DID YOU KNOW:

- Bipolar disorder is the leading cause of suicide in the country.

- Sufferers are more likely to seek support and treatment when they're depressed than when they are manic.

- Fewer than one third of the people who have the illness are ever treated for it.

- Writers Virginia Woolf, Leo Tolstoy, and Robert Lowell, and leaders Napoleon Bonaparte and Winston Churchill suffered from bipolar disorder.

- Bipolar disorder affects both men and women equally. However, first episodes for men tend to be manic, whereas in women they are generally depressive.

- Nearly 50 percent of all bipolar disorder patients have at least one parent with a mood disorder.

- Women often show their first signs of bipolar disorder during a postpartum period.

LEARN THE CRUCIAL FACTS, PLUS THE LATEST INFORMATION ON NEW TREATMENTS, ALTERNATIVE THERAPIES, SCIENTIFIC BREAKTHROUGHS, AND MUCH MORE IN . . .

WHY AM I UP? WHY AM I DOWN?

The Dell Guides for Mental Health

If You Think You Have Depression

If You Think You Have Panic Disorder

If You Think You Have an Eating Disorder

If You Think You Have Seasonal Affective Disorder

If You Think You Have a Sleep Disorder

Why Am I Up, Why Am I Down? Understanding Bipolar Disorder

Why Does Everything Have to Be Perfect? Understanding Obsessive-Compulsive Disorder

Why Am I Still so Afraid? Understanding Post-Traumatic Stress Disorder

Why Am I Up, Why Am I Down?

Understanding Bipolar Disorder

Roger Granet, M.D.
and
Elizabeth Ferber

A Dell Mental Health Guide
Series Editor: Roger Granet, M.D.

A DELL BOOK

Published by
Dell Publishing
a division of
Random House, Inc.
1540 Broadway
New York, New York 10036

Dell books may be purchased for business or promotional use or for special sales. For information please write to: Special Markets Department, Random House, Inc., 1540 Broadway, New York, N.Y. 10036.

Dell® is a registered trademark of Random House, Inc., and the colophon is a trademark of Random House, Inc.

ISBN: 0-440-23465-4

Designed by Donna Sinisgalli

Printed in the United States of America

Published simultaneously in Canada

August 1999

10 9 8 7 6 5 4 3 2 1

OPM

Acknowledgments

Thanks to . . .

Those people with bipolar disorder and their loved ones who have the courage to live life more fully.

Judith Riven, whose encouragement was a major factor in the completion of this book.

Laurie Martin, Lesley Meisoll, and Clifford Taylor, M.D., in Dr. Granet's office for their constant insight and support.

Janis Vallely for making the call.

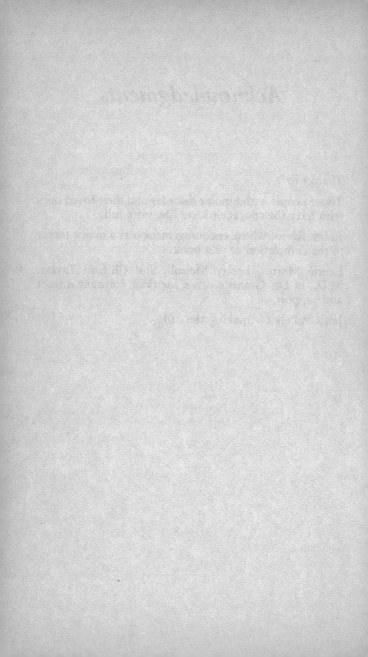

Contents

Foreword

The beauty of the world has two edges,
one of laughter, one of anguish,
cutting the heart asunder.

Few writers capture the inherent paradox of manic-depressive illness, currently referred to as bipolar disorder, as poignantly as Virginia Woolf. Struggling with both her muse and her demons, Woolf conveys through her words the complexity of living with bipolar disorder. Anyone who has experienced the manic "highs" and depressive "lows" of the illness understands how both laughter and anguish can define the condition. Tragically for Woolf, she lived during a time of limited insight into the disorder and few available treatments. Fortunately, those with bipolar disorder today have a host of treatment options that combine to lessen the potentially devastating effects of the illness.

In most societies throughout history, it has been both natural and acceptable to experience a medical illness. Those who have heart attacks or diabetes are viewed as "normal" people who just happen to have a problem affecting an organ system of the body. Yet, when that organ system happens to be the brain, those with the illness are suddenly viewed as abnormal and often spoken about in pejorative whispers.

Why such a dichotomy? Fear, lack of knowledge, and outdated perceptions remain the cornerstones of bias against mental illness. And when the words "bipolar disorder" and "lithium" are mentioned, people are even more apt to show prejudice.

The irony of this dichotomy is that bipolar disorder

is really no different from any other disease. Having a disease simply implies an interruption in the function of any significant part of the body. Rather than arteries obstructed by cholesterol or a malfunctioning pancreas unable to produce insulin, bipolar disorder is an illness of the brain. It is a disorder that temporarily alters normal and healthy brain activity.

Adding to the irony is the fact that with modern diagnostic techniques and rapid advances in genetics, biology, psychology, and sociology, bipolar disorder is, in many ways, more treatable and less progressive than either cardiac disease or diabetes.

Bipolar disorder is an illness that affects not only individuals but entire families. This book is for anyone with questions or concerns regarding the condition, about which most people have little knowledge. Adding to the mystery and confusion surrounding the disorder is the fact that it is no longer referred to as manic-depressive illness or manic depression, but is now called bipolar disorder. The former title is at least self-explanatory in that it describes the extremes of mood a person experiences.

Considering that there are more than two million people in the United States currently diagnosed with bipolar disorder, there is a great need to educate and inform. Families, friends, and colleagues of those with the illness, not to mention the general public, are best served with the kind of simple, straightforward information this book aims to provide.

For decades, bipolar disorder has taken second seat to its more popular cousin, unipolar depression. Thanks to a revolution in diagnosis and treatment for unipolar depression, today few people have to live with its often debilitating effects. Bipolar disorder, on the other hand, is harder for doctors to treat, is more challenging for patients to live with, and presents a greater diagnostic enigma than does unipolar depression. Neglecting the severity of bipolar disorder can have tragic implications. This illness is the leading cause of suicide in the country.

Since the development of a rigorous and reliable set of criteria for defining bipolar disorder, patients receive treatment sooner than ever before. In clear language and comprehensible terms, the criteria for a bipolar diagnosis is presented in the early chapters of this book. The basic structure of the illness involves alternating episodes of mild to severe depression and mania. The milder form of mania is more commonly referred to as hypomania. To meet the criteria for either bipolar I (episodes of depression and mania) or bipolar II (episodes of depression and hypomania), patients must present a very specific set of symptoms for a designated period of time.

The most telling of symptoms is an alteration in mood, because depression, sadness and despondency, and hopelessness are the predominant factors. Additionally, patients usually suffer an overall lack of energy as well as a lack of interest in formerly pleasurable activities, while having to cope with diminished concentration and changes in sleep patterns. Mania involves an excessively elevated or elated mood along with rapid speech, increased energy, and racing thoughts. Occasionally, patients experience delusions and can become psychotic. Patients who are hypomanic tend to experience an excess of energy coupled with overly optimistic feelings and a decreased need for sleep and food. Making the task of diagnosing bipolar disorder that much more complicated for doctors is the fact that many other factors and medical conditions can induce symptoms that mimic the illness.

Misdiagnosing a patient who has bipolar disorder can result in the disorder's most severe consequence, suicide. In the past, little could be done to prevent a patient from taking his or her own life. Psychiatrists, psychologists, and social workers base a newfound optimism on the accumulation of clinical experience and the development of technological advances used to diagnose and treat not only bipolar disorder but psychiatric illnesses as a whole.

Recent biological, psychological, and sociological

studies have already begun to yield hope-inspiring results and refined diagnostic criteria. Using the newly
designated subgroups of bipolar I, II, and III (the last
being an unofficial diagnosis), experts are able to offer
more specific treatments for the illness based on actual
symptoms. In addition to an extensive physical and psychological examination, doctors now use family histories as an aid in making a diagnosis of bipolar disorder.
As experts begin to isolate suspected genes, the case for
a strong genetic component that passes the disorder
from one relative to another becomes increasingly valid.
Children of bipolar parents often show early signs of
mood instability and have a greater than 50 percent
chance of developing the disorder.

Experts now believe bipolar disorder to have as
strong a biological component as any of the psychiatric
illnesses. Studies in brain chemistry that control mood
reveal a disturbance in neurotransmitter activity and the
chemical messengers of the brain. Abnormal functioning of certain brain chemicals, like gaba-aminobutyric
acid (GABA), impede crucial operating mechanisms in
the brain. Use of cutting-edge radiological techniques,
including positron emission tomography (PET scans)
and single photon emission computerized tomography
(SPECT scans), reveal the specific areas of the brain that
correspond to the illness, and may help pinpoint its
physiological causes.

Refining the techniques that shed light on the causes
of bipolar disorder allow experts to develop treatments
tailored to the specific needs of patients. In the past,
lithium was the only medication available to bipolar
patients, but today there are a host of medication options. Anticonvulsants, predominantly used in the treatment of seizure disorders like epilepsy, are now in the
forefront of bipolar medications. Depakote is probably
the most popular choice for the acute and maintenance
phases of the illness, with Tegretol (pending FDA approval) not far behind. Other anticonvulsants, including Neurontin and Lamictal, are also showing excellent
results.

Antidepressants are now flooding the market, with more than two dozen available for treatment as of this writing. When prescribing antidepressants for bipolar patients, doctors must use extreme caution so as not to induce mania. Close monitoring and open communication among patient, doctor, and family should prevent swings into mania, but the possibility is always present. Modern antidepressants, overall, are far more effective and have fewer side effects than their earlier counterparts developed in the late 1960s. Currently in development are a series of blood tests that would allow scientists to determine which antidepressant would be most effective for a specific patient.

Perhaps no procedure has been more maligned by the general public than electroconvulsive therapy (ECT). It is without a doubt one of the most misunderstood treatments for both unipolar depression and bipolar disorder. However, contemporary ECT is effectve and safe, and it is commonly used by doctors for patients who cannot tolerate or have become resistant to medication. Currently both repetitive transcranial magnetic stimulation (rTMS) and even a fish oil component, known as omega-3 fatty acids, may show promise for combating episodes of bipolar disorder with almost no side effects.

There is little question that bipolar disorder is a biologically rooted illness. However, this does not diminish the complex emotions that patients experience when they learn that they have the disorder, let alone when they begin to cope with its effects on their lives. In addition, the devastating psychological consequences of both depressive and manic episodes on individuals and their families cannot be ignored. Therefore, a host of psychotherapeutic techniques are available to bipolar sufferers that are alternately effective depending on the patient's current state. Even though some therapies are more productive for bipolar disorder than others, a discussion of all the available techniques is presented in chapter 5. Perhaps the most useful types of therapies for bipolar patients are the ones that help them cope with their behavior and fluctuating mood on a day-to-day basis. The most promising is cognitive behavioral therapy, which attempts to redirect a patient's negative thoughts and behavior patterns toward a more positive, integrated outlook.

Most essential to bipolar patients and their families is psychoeducation—where they learn the realities of the illness and how to cope with them. The death of a loved one, switching jobs, the birth of a child, divorce, or moving to a new city can all be stressful enough to induce a bipolar episode. Those with the illness, and their immediate circle of intimates, must learn the symptoms of incipient mania and depressive episodes in order to prevent full-blown episodes. Anticipating events or situations that create stress and anxiety in a person's life is part of managing the illness. People with bipolar disorder often have to lead lives with lower levels of stimulation and pressure to function normally. This may include working in a less stressful office setting and avoiding chemical substances like caffeine and alcohol.

The brain is a precious, complicated organ, yet in essence it is just another of the body's organs. We can hope, considering the wealth of knowledge we now have about psychiatric disorders, that long-held prejudices and stigmatizing biases may finally be put to rest. In particular, the state of modern diagnosis and treatment are powerful reasons to be optimistic, especially since most people with bipolar disorder lead active, healthy, and fulfilling lives.

It is time to stop whispering about bipolar disorder. Effective diagnoses and treatments are available if we speak out loud, offering hope and healing for those with bipolar disorder and their loved ones.

Roger Granet, M.D., F.A.P.A.
Clinical Professor of Psychiatry
Cornell University Medical College

Morristown, New Jersey, 1998

Chapter 1

BIPOLAR DISORDER: DEFINITIONS AND OVERVIEW

It often feels as if we live in a world of endless contradictions. The more we work, the more money we make, yet ironically, the less time we have to enjoy it. Another classic example, according to Pentagon officials, is that the more bombs we build, the safer we will ostensibly be. How do we handle these and life's other fundamental contradictions? We pay attention to events around us, we continue with our daily tasks, and we simply hope for the best. When it comes to life's inherent contradictions, the world of mental illness is no exception, claiming as its own a disease that truly embodies the meaning of the word "opposite": The disease is bipolar disorder, formerly and more commonly known as manic-depressive illness. Bipolar disorder can be likened to the painted face of a circus clown: at once robustly joyous and at other times profoundly sad.

The clown analogy, which is commonly used when describing bipolar disorder, is an apt one, but it does not begin to address the complexity of the illness. The disease is perhaps one of the most mysterious and understudied illnesses in the field of mental health. It is estimated that 11 to 15 million Americans suffer from some form of mood disorder, whether it be major depressive disorder, dysthymic disorder, bipolar I disorder, bipolar II disorder, or cyclothymic disorder. Of the afflicted, at least 2 million people, or 0.4 to 1.6 percent of the population in the United States, experience the "highs" and "lows" of bipolar disorder.

Bipolar disorder is differentiated from other forms of depression by its periods of intense mania and/or hypomania. Sufferers experience black and hopeless moods of depression, but also euphoric feelings of hypomania and often psychotic periods of mania. In between episodes of depression and mania, patients may experience periods of balanced moods, where they feel relatively normal or "euthymic." A person may, for example, be manic for three to six months, euthymic for six months after that, and then depressed for six to nine months. As we come to understand more about this illness that takes its toll on spousal, familial, and other interpersonal relationships, we know that far more people have lived with bipolar disorder than was formerly thought. A devastating reality of bipolar disorder is that fewer than one-third of those who have the illness are ever treated for it. For a host of complex reasons, bipolar disorder is often misdiagnosed or simply goes undetected, sometimes at the expense of the sufferer's life. We do know that at least 15 percent of those who have bipolar disorder take their own lives, that men who suffer from the illness are more likely to commit suicide than women, and that these people take their own lives most often during a depressive episode.

Often, describing just the technical aspects of a disease like bipolar disorder tells only half of the story. Without personal anecdotes and case studies the material can seem dry, removed, and not terribly relevant. This is why, throughout the book, we will be presenting stories and histories of individuals coping with the disease.

Has bipolar disorder existed for a long time?

One of the great mysteries of bipolar disorder is its etiology, or cause. We will explore this subject at greater length in chapter 3, but it may help to address some of the issues here. There is a substantial amount of evidence that mood disorders, including bipolar, have existed since antiquity. Many ancient documents, including the Old Testament story of King Saul and Ajax's suicide in Homer's *Iliad*, describe serious depressive episodes. Even the father of medicine, the Greek physician Hippocrates, noted both mania and melancholia when discussing certain mental abnormalities. The alternating moods of bipolar disorder were not formally recorded until about the mid–nineteenth century, when two French doctors, Jules Falret and Jules G. F. Baillarger, noted that several patients showed both depressed and manic symptoms over a period of time. It was not until 1882 that the German psychiatrist Karl Kahlbaum coined the term *cyclothymia,* which describes depression and mania as parts of the same disease. In 1899, psychiatrist Emil Kraepelin, using the knowledge of his French and German predecessors, established a criterion for a manic-depressive psychosis that psychiatrists still use for diagnosing bipolar I today.

If we look back to some of the more celebrated figures of the past three hundred years, it is clear that writers Virginia Woolf, Leo Tolstoy, and Robert Lowell and leaders Napoleon Bonaparte and Winston Churchill all may have suffered from bipolar disorder. Woolf discussed her experience with fluctuating moods through characters in many of her books and clearly struggled with the illness all her life. In 1941, her depression became too much to bear and she committed suicide, cutting short a stellar literary career. Formerly, there was little insight into what caused the alternating moods of these outstanding individuals, nor was there any legitimate treatment to offer them relief.

What is the current understanding of bipolar disorder?

At present, there is an ever-increasing amount of research into the triggers and causes of bipolar disorder, yet there is still much to be learned. Some researchers have tried to divide the causative factors into biological, genetic, and psychosocial components, but these components become difficult to pinpoint as the three constantly interact with each other. Recently, scientists have found that bipolar disorder may stem from multiple genes. Researchers have discovered new sites on five chromosomes that may contain genes that predispose an individual to the illness. The reports are still provisional, but they point in the direction of real progress in an understanding of the disorder.

If you are predisposed to develop bipolar disorder, what is it that triggers the first episode of the illness or the reappearance of symptoms?

For Janet, a thirty-six-year-old mother of one, the birth of her second child reignited symptoms of bipolar disorder that had appeared four years prior in the form of a hypomanic episode. Janet had taken Depakote, an anticonvulsant used as a mood stabilizer for bipolar mania and sometimes depression, but had stopped taking it during pregnancy. She was concerned about possible birth defects. Two months after the birth of her second child, Janet began to experience the "blues" on a daily basis and noticed the onset of an irritable mood. "I was able to fall asleep, but I woke up frequently during the night and I began to lose my appetite," she recalls. "I felt guilty about not wanting to breast-feed the new baby and about not feeling any connection to the children. I was generally overwhelmed by everything from the children to the housework." It was not long before she started having thoughts of suicide.

Fortunately, Janet realized that her symptoms were beyond transient blues, and after talking it over with her husband, Bill, she consulted her psychologist. "Bill and I met with the psychologist," Janet says, "and he confirmed that I was experiencing a postpartum depression that had triggered symptoms of my bipolar disorder. He immediately referred me to a psychiatrist." Because the psychiatrist knew of Janet's hypomanic history, he put her on the antidepressant Paxil with

Depakote to avoid a swing from depression to mania. Within three weeks, Janet noticed a marked improvement in her mood, sleep patterns, and feelings toward her children. Her family and friends had provided crucial support by cooking meals and taking care of housework when she felt she needed rest. Thankfully, Janet's doctor helped her understand the roots of her depression, that it was tied to her loss of autonomy owing to the new baby and other family responsibilities. In six weeks, Janet was back to baseline functioning and needed only to continue on the Depakote for four months to prevent any impending episodes.

While a bipolar episode can be triggered by a specific life event, as in Janet's case, the disease can also appear autonomously without any apparent instigator. Because bipolar episodes are not always preceded by a stressful life event, they often go undetected by family and friends. In addition, patients tend to deny and try to conceal their symptoms. The illness can also mask itself as another problem—for example, drug or alcohol abuse or poor work performance—thus making it much more difficult to recognize and treat. Unlike sickle-cell anemia or Tay-Sachs disease, which both occur in specific ethnic and racial groups, bipolar disorder does not prevail in any one cultural circle. Because bipolar disorder, like other mental illnesses, crosses all ethnic and racial boundaries and does not discriminate, the task of identifying the disease is quite challenging. The only variable that researchers have found is that clinicians tend to underdiagnose patients of a different ethnic and racial group from their own, as is true of most other medical conditions.

How is bipolar disorder treated?

There have been significant and encouraging breakthroughs in the treatment of bipolar disorder, with researchers focusing not only on the critical area of medications, but also on psychoeducation and psychosocial therapy. In chapters 5 and 6 we will examine how current and past medications and therapies have helped those with bipolar disorder navigate their lives. Formerly, lithium was the drug of choice for all bipolar patients, but it often brought with it debilitating and potentially life-altering side effects. With the advent of a host of new drug treatments and technological advances in brain imaging, which clinicians use for diagnosis, a patient's options have increased significantly. Medication is imperative for treating the illness in its acute phase, maintaining stability, and preventing recurrence of this potentially chronic condition. Mental health professionals generally agree, however, that learning about the disorder and its potentially devastating effects on a person's life, coupled with an ongoing relationship with a psychiatrist or other mental health professional is also vital.

Are there particular difficulties in treating or working with bipolar patients?

Perhaps the most frustrating aspect of treating bipolar disorder is not limited to medications or psychiatric therapies, but to a patient's frequent refusal to comply with a doctor's orders. In a hypomanic or manic phase, sufferers often deny the fact that they are acting abnormally and refuse to take their medications. While some feel that they just plain do not need them, many view medication as a hindrance in their grand scheme to reach glorious destinies.

Occasionally, in a manic state, patients can become aggressive and violent toward family and doctors, making it difficult and dangerous to work with them. Jonathan, who was diagnosed with bipolar disorder at age twenty-two, began taking maintenance medication to block a return of symptoms after an acute phase of mania. Once his mood stabilized, he decided he no longer needed his medication and discontinued his doctor's recommended treatment. When symptoms reappeared, Jonathan once again had to begin a regimen of medications that took several months to take effect. The lapse cost him a semester of graduate school.

In a depressed phase, patients may feel too hopeless and initially lack the energy to seek out or continue medication and therapy. The principal goals of contemporary treatment are to diagnose accurately a person's condition, stabilize them after an acute manic or depressed episode, and begin a treatment that includes medication and psychotherapy. Additionally, clinicians must always try to ensure the safety of a patient in either phase of the disorder. The therapist must constantly strive to properly assess any suicide risk when a patient is depressed, or gauge when a patient is endangering himself through reckless behavior when manic. To enable them to make appropriate decisions, patients and their families need education about the course of bipolar disorder. All of their lives are affected.

Knowledge about treatment will help sufferers stick to a plan once they have returned to functioning at a normal level, commonly referred to as "baseline." More specifically, baseline is the goal that patients and doctors strive for when creating a medication and therapy regime after either a manic or depressive episode. As we will see, one of the most important periods for patients, their families, and their doctors to work together is the time between episodes of mania and depression, when a person is able to function without the debilitating symptoms of the disease.

How is bipolar depression different from unipolar depression?

When someone mentions that she is feeling depressed, most of us can identify and empathize with her. We know what it feels like to be down in the dumps, feeling blue, somewhat hopeless about our lives, or just plain sad. Many people experience depression after a specific life event triggers an emotional response—for example, the death of a loved one or the birth of a child. However, most people recover from their depressed feelings without any serious disruption of their everyday lives. For those who suffer from a major depressive disorder, this is not the case. Often they cannot shake their feelings of hopelessness and worthlessness, and their lives are affected as a result. When depression persists, interfering with family relationships, work, sleep patterns, and the ability to carry out daily tasks, it is imperative that the sufferer talk to someone about it, whether a family member, friend, or medical professional.

The feelings and characteristics of bipolar and unipolar depressive conditions are, for the most part, the same. The length of time of a depression may differ, but your mood is affected in the same way. Researchers are currently conducting studies on how the two forms might differ more significantly, but there is no definitive data at the moment. It is hoped that finding greater distinctions will lead to bipolar depression being treated more specifically vis-à-vis the disorder's other symptoms. *If You Think You Have Depression*, another book in the Dell Guides for Mental Health, offers a more detailed discussion of depression in general and how it affects people's lives.

What is hypomania and mania?

Initially, mania can feel like a door that opens onto all of life's grand possibilities. Kay Redfield Jamison, a well-known authority on bipolar disorder and the author of *An Unquiet Mind: A Memoir of Moods and Madness*, describes her early and seemingly mild manic moods as "intoxicating states that gave rise to great personal pleasure, an incomparable flow of thoughts, and a ceaseless energy." The alteration of mood may reach almost a fever pitch, the patient functioning at an almost superhuman level; this state is commonly referred to by mental health professionals as "hypomanic." Unfortunately, hypomanic states may deteriorate into increasingly irresponsible and irrational behavior, including a grandiose and often distorted sense of self, poor judgment and impulsiveness, excessive spending, and sexual promiscuity. As the person reels further and further toward mania, they begin to need less sleep and food, and may begin to experience delusions (false beliefs) and, less frequently, hallucinations (false perceptions).

It is crucial for family members and friends to be able to identify these symptoms so that the patient is diagnosed and treated before a potentially life-threatening situation occurs. There are several steps that relatives and friends can take to determine whether or not their child or friend is experiencing a hypomanic or manic episode. If you suspect that someone might be having a hypomanic episode, the best thing to do is observe his behavior:

- Does he appear more energetic and elated than usual?
- Has he been staying awake later and longer than usual?
- Has he been skipping meals and appearing less interested in food?
- Has he been spending what seems like an excessive amount of money recently?
- Has he been working longer hours than usual or studying harder?
- Is he more comfortable asking people out on dates or, if you can possibly find out, is he more sexually promiscuous?
- Has he become more irritable and aggressive when asked about the change in his behavior?

It can be rather difficult to ask direct questions to a person who is in a hypomanic or a manic condition. If he is experiencing hypomania for the first time, he probably will not be able to discern that anything is unusual about his behavior. If he becomes manic, his sense of himself will probably be distorted to such an extent that hospitalization is required.

What can someone do to intercede when a friend or family member seems endangered?

Getting help can seem like a daunting task for the family and friends of a person with bipolar disorder, but as symptoms get worse over time, it is prudent not to wait long before acting. The following are some initial steps:

- Contact any friends who you know have had experience with mental health professionals, like psychologists or psychiatrists. Ask your friends for a referral.
- Call a mental health professional you know and ask her if the symptoms that you have observed could indicate something serious.
- Ask family members if there is a history of any mental disorders in the family. Having information about a person's history is very important when trying to determine a diagnosis.
- Phone a national mental health organization, like the National Depressive and Manic Depressive Association (NDMDA), and ask them whom to contact.
- Alert health services at a school if a student begins to exhibit unusual behavior.

David, a usually mild-mannered twenty-year-old college junior majoring in biology and with plans to attend medical school, was lucky that his roommates decided to call health services when he began staying up late, propositioning women, studying obsessively, and believing that he had discovered a new model for a molecular formula. David's parents soon arrived, and they all met with a psychologist at the school's health services office who referred them to a psychiatrist, who is a medical doctor. After making a full psychological examination and taking a medical and family history, the psychiatrist determined that David should be put on lithium and Klonopin (an antianxiety agent) to relieve his manic symptoms. The two medications worked well in combination, and in two weeks David settled down and began twice-weekly sessions with a therapist. Thanks to the support of friends, family, and his health care professional, David returned to baseline functioning in only six weeks.

Fortunately, David's unusual symptoms were recognized and he was able to seek treatment. Often this is not the case with an initial onset of bipolar disorder with manic symptoms. Friends and family do not always take the initiative; sufferers can be quite resistant; and the disorder is often misdiagnosed by doctors, like internists and gynecologists, who are not familiar with its symptoms. If a hypomanic condition continues toward mania, hospitalization and inpatient services are often required. It is common for manic patients to abuse drugs, alcohol, and other chemical substances that may endanger their lives and make it difficult for professionals to treat them. Determining whether manic symptoms are the result of substance abuse or are actually attributable to bipolar disorder is a great diagnostic challenge. Important information about a person's condition is often impossible to retrieve by the time he or she is admitted to the hospital in a manic state.

What is the difference between bipolar I, II, and III?

Understanding the complexity of bipolar disorder means being able to distinguish between the different layers of the illness. Mental health professionals now classify the disorder into several different categories, thus ensuring that every patient is treated for his or her specific symptoms. The *Diagnostic and Statistical Manual of Mental Disorders—Fourth Edition,* or *DSM-IV* (American Psychiatric Association, 1994), generally accepted as the definitive source on mental illness, recognizes two official diagnoses for bipolar disorder (I and II), but a third is often unofficially discussed. The authors of *DSM-IV* have extensively researched bipolar disorder and have obtained reliable criteria for the following descriptions:

- Bipolar I disorder is distinguished by a person having one or more manic or mixed episodes (a period of time lasting at least one week where a person meets the criteria for both a manic and depressive episode nearly every day) and usually a major depression.

- Bipolar II disorder sufferers have one or more major depressive episodes and at least one hypomanic episode. Bipolar II appears to affect 0.5 percent of the adult population over a lifetime.

- Bipolar III (currently being investigated by researchers) is an unofficial distinction made when a patient suffers from a general depression but becomes manic owing to antidepressant medication. Usually, a family history of bipolar disorder is present in patients with bipolar III, and it occurs most often in young women, with an abrupt onset.

- One other diagnosis in the bipolar family is cyclothymic disorder, where a patient suffers numerous hypomanic and mild depressive episodes over a period lasting at least two years.

Researchers have found that bipolar I affects men and women in equal numbers, yet for some reason bipolar II is more common in women. Among racial and ethnic groups, the prevalence of both illnesses is about the same. Bipolar disorder is not a disorder of the rich or the poor per se, but an illness that is closely tied to a person's family history and life events. However, socioeconomics may play a role in whether a person has access to treatment. In fact, the illness does have a higher-than-average incidence among more affluent individuals, but this may relate to greater availability of therapy and health care in general for the rich. All members of society, it appears, can develop the disease.

How are bipolar disorders different from other mood disorders?

The bipolar disorders distinguish themselves from other illnesses within the mood disorder family by having as a central component hypomanic and manic episodes. Compared to many other types of illnesses, mood disorders are common human afflictions. By some estimates 12 to 15 percent of women and 8 to 10 percent of men in America will struggle with some variation of a mood disturbance over the course of a lifetime. Generally, the mental health community divides mood disorders into depressive disorders—which, as discussed previously, are unipolar depressions—the bipolar disorders, and two disorders that are based on either general medical conditions (e.g., hypothyroidism, anemia) or substance abuse (e.g., alcohol and drug use). For the last two, clinicians are faced with the challenge of determining whether an individual's mood disturbance is caused by a condition other than true bipolar disorder.

Non–bipolar mood disorders include:

- *Major depressive disorder,* where a person is seriously depressed for at least two weeks and exhibits several other symptoms of a major depression, like loss of sleep and appetite. Those suffering from a major depression of this kind generally need the help of a professional before they can find relief from the disorder.

- *Dysthymic disorder* is a milder form of depression that lasts at least two years in adults and one in children and adolescents. Historically, it has been referred to as "depressive personality" or "neurotic depression."

- *Depressive disorder not otherwise specified* is a classification used by clinicians for purposes of identifying disorders that have depressive features but do not meet the criteria for a full-blown, major depression.

- *Mood disorder due to a general medical condition* is a necessary classification when trying to determine a diagnosis, because several medical conditions, such as hypothyroidism, present symptoms that are strikingly similar to mood disorders. In chapter 2, we will

examine other conditions that cause mood disturbances.

- *Substance-induced mood disorder* is generally
caused by a person's use of illicit or prescription
drugs or alcohol. Thousands of drugs are known to
cause depression as a side effect, and alcohol is a
depressant. Informing your health care provider
about any chemical substances that you are taking,
prescribed and otherwise, is imperative if you are
trying to uncover a cause for your mood disorder.

Who is affected by bipolar disorder?

Just as bipolar disorder does not discriminate based on
a person's race or ethnicity, it also does not particularly pay attention to a person's age. The illness has
been diagnosed in children as young as five and six,
but, thankfully, it is not common in this age group.
Clinicians sometimes understandably confuse bipolar
disorder with attention deficit hyperactivity disorder
(ADHD), since both illnesses present themselves with
similar sets of symptoms. Properly diagnosing a child
with one of these two disorders is necessary if she is to
get the proper treatment. Since 1980, adults and children have been diagnosed with bipolar disorder using
the same criteria. However, because there are so many
variables when it comes to truly uncovering what a
child is suffering from, some special rules now apply.
Clinicians must take into account the developmental
age of the child and how that affects the expression of
certain symptoms. For example, normal behavior in
children may occasionally resemble a hypomanic episode.

Do young children have specific symptoms that parents, teachers, and doctors should look for?

In young children, identifying episodes of mania and
depression is often very difficult. Bipolar disorder can
present itself in a variety of ways, including a course of

behavior that gets better and then worsens over time. Some of the signs to look for are disruptive behavior in school, moodiness, irritability, sleep difficulties, impulsive acts, hyperactivity, explosive anger followed by feelings of guilt, and a noted inability to concentrate. A comprehensive study on the prevalence of bipolar disorder in children has not yet been conducted, making it difficult to generalize on diagnostic and treatment methods. For adolescents, the prevalence appears to be the same as that for adults, ranging from 0.6 to 1.1 percent. However, studies of adolescents also show distinct periods of symptoms that appear to be hypomanic without fulfilling the criteria for bipolar disorder. In other words, an adolescent may have been symptomatic for several years but the illness has gone undetected and untreated. According to the results of a membership survey of the National Depressive and Manic Depressive Association (NDMDA), 59 percent of responding adults reported the onset of bipolar disorder during childhood and adolescence. Looking for the signs of a child at risk begins with noticing:

- sudden swings in mood, whether from positive to negative
- increased irritability and disinterest in activities
- a family history of mood disorders
- delusions
- psychomotor retardation
- trouble sleeping

With most adolescents, it is also a good idea to test for drugs if symptoms of hypomanic or manic behavior suddenly appear.

When does bipolar disorder usually manifest in adults?

Bipolar disorder in adults has a prevalence of about 1 percent, with equal dominance in both men and women. First episodes for men tend to be manic rather than depressive, whereas in women they are generally depressive. Many patients actually experience several bouts of depression before ever having a manic episode. Most people experience their first symptoms of bipolar disorder, whether depressive or manic, between the ages of nineteen and twenty-four, averaging out in the early twenties. Tragically, there is usually a five- to ten-year interval between the onset of the actual illness and a patient's first treatment or hospitalization.

A diagnosis at age fifty is certainly not unheard of, and some individuals are in fact first diagnosed in their retirement years. For those who develop bipolar disorder over the age of sixty, there is likely to be a strong family history of the illness. Additionally, the symptoms of the disorder are more likely to be associated with a medical condition, including cerebral vascular ailments, than a specific mood disturbance.

Profiling of those who have bipolar disorder reveals that more divorced and single people have the illness, possibly reflecting the disease's early onset and resulting relationship difficulties. The disorder also appears to be more common in those who did not attend college than in those who did, but again this could reflect an early diagnosis and subsequent problems.

Can bipolar disorder ever be cured?

Bipolar disorder is often a chronic illness, and it can almost always be treated with great effort on the part of the patient and therapist, but thus far it cannot be cured. Currently, most psychiatrists present bipolar disorder to their patients in terms of how to improve the quality of their lives by learning how to cope with their illness rather than focusing on a cure. It is recurrent in 90 percent of individuals who have only a single manic episode, and nearly 60 to 70 percent of all manic episodes occur before or after a major depression. Formerly, many in the psychiatric community viewed bipolar disorder as mild compared to the severity of a disease like schizophrenia, but in reality, the illness exacts no less of a toll on a person's life.

What is the present outlook for those diagnosed with bipolar disorder?

The economic cost of mood disorders is estimated to exceed $40 billion in the United States each year, an onus far greater than that of heart disease. The high economic price to society is compounded by the social cost of drug and alcohol addiction, a common consequence of mood disorders, if they go untreated. Fortunately, society is becoming more aware of the issues surrounding these debilitating and sometimes life-threatening disorders. Chapter 4 explains how you can find and receive help from resources within your own family, community, and hospital support groups. National organizations, like the National Depressive and Manic Depressive Association (NDMDA), provide excellent referral networks and places to begin on the path toward a happier and healthier existence.

In addition to the pharmacological and psychotherapeutic treatments discussed in chapters 5 and 6, chapter 7 discusses adjunctive therapies, like electroconvulsive therapy (ECT) and sleep deprivation, with both positive and negative aspects for bipolar patients.

Currently, bipolar disorder is an affliction that sufferers must cope with over a lifetime. In the final chapter, chapter 8, we will focus on coping skills and goal establishment. With adherence to a manageable medication regime, support from family, friends, groups, and skillful and empathic therapists, bipolar disorder does not have to dominate your every waking moment. It can simply become just another aspect of who you are.

Chapter 2

SYMPTOMS AND DIAGNOSIS OF BIPOLAR DISORDER

Why is bipolar disorder so often misdiagnosed or undetected?

With the benefit of hindsight, it is obvious that bipolar disorder has been around for centuries. Unfortunately, due to a lack of awareness about the illness, those who suffered from it throughout history rarely found any relief from their fluctuating moods. Today, there is certainly more understanding and knowledge surrounding the disease, but all too often it still goes undetected owing to the public's lack of knowledge about the disease. According to some reports, nearly half of all bipolar disorder sufferers are misdiagnosed, and go untreated, for several years. This tragic reality is even more devastating because an early diagnosis can make all the difference for an effective treatment.

One study of mentally ill patients who were admitted to a two-week inpatient program revealed that only thirty of fifty patients with bipolar disorder were properly diagnosed before entering the treatment facility. The thirty patients who had been diagnosed with the disorder prior to admission had all received the diagnosis within a year of seeking help. Unfortunately for the twenty patients who were misdiagnosed, up to eight years had passed from the time they first sought help to the time they were finally diagnosed with bipolar disorder. This study suggests that if you are not diagnosed with bipolar disorder right away, you will probably spend several years with a mistaken diagnosis of, for example, unipolar depression. Wasting that much time on a misdiagnosis is extremely harmful to a patient with bipolar disorder. Tragically, the illness often worsens over time and can sometimes become resistant to treatment.

How will a doctor know if I have bipolar disorder versus a major depressive disorder?

Your doctor will first determine if you do in fact have a major depressive disorder before investigating further. A comprehensive list of all the symptoms for a major depressive disorder is presented later in this chapter. Once she has decided that you do in fact meet the criteria for a major depressive disorder, the next step is to discover if you have bipolar disorder. She will do this by trying to find out whether you have ever had an episode of hypomania or mania. There are several criteria you must meet before she can establish a diagnosis for true bipolar disorder. Patients are not always able to establish whether they have had prior episodes of hypomania and mania. In fact, probably about half of all bipolar patients will not tell their doctors they have had a manic episode even during a careful interview.

Your doctor may want to consult a family member to better help her establish whether you have ever been hypomanic or manic in the past. Family members can be very helpful once they have been given a full list of symptoms for hypomania and mania, and are often very reliable sources. In addition, apprising them of the signs of bipolar disorder is instrumental in preventing the onset and escalation of future episodes.

How can I tell whether I have a clinical depression and not just the "blues"?

Most of us experience the "blues" several times during a lifetime. When someone we love moves away or when we lose a job, it is normal to feel down, sad, and somewhat hopeless. However, as time goes by, our daily activities distract us from the emotional pain, our mood brightens, and we begin to feel good again. If a mental health professional determines that you have a clinical depression, however, you are not able to shake off the blues so easily. You need help to understand why you have no interest in your work, family, or hobbies. Sometimes psychotherapy and medication are needed to ensure that you can continue to function normally. Whether you are feeling sad or are suffering from a severe clinical depression, it is always useful to seek advice and help. If friends and family are not enough, contact a professional.

How can I determine if I have a serious clinical depression?

Clinical depressions have a very distinct set of symptoms that make them easily recognizable to clinicians. Once you have determined that you need the advice of a professional, he will ask you a number of questions about your mental state. The clinician must figure out how disruptive the depression has been to your life before making a diagnosis. He must assess a number of variables to gauge the seriousness of your condition. These include intensity, duration, and the number of symptoms you are experiencing. Generally, clinicians consider two or three symptoms that do not dramatically interfere with your life a mild case of depression. If there are more symptoms and they last for weeks at a time, you probably meet the criteria for a serious depressive episode.

David, a successful real estate lawyer, finally went to see a psychiatrist after eight weeks of depressed mood, loss of interest in work, insomnia, and lack of appetite. He told the doctor, "I used to love going to work. Now I can barely get out of bed in the morning." David's doctor determined after additional questions that he did meet the criteria for a major depressive disorder. The doctor prescribed a course of antidepressants and weekly psychotherapy sessions.

As a general rule, the more disruptive the symptoms to your life, the more serious your depression. If you choose to examine your symptoms one by one, keep in mind that major depressions express themselves through multiple symptoms, not singular ones.

How can I tell if my symptoms are getting worse?

Symptoms of depression can begin rather mildly and then escalate without warning. If you think you may have a major depression, note the symptoms and track their progression. For example, consider loss of appetite, which can begin with a mild lack of interest in food. Soon you start to skip breakfast, claiming that you are not hungry in the morning. Lunch is next to go, and before you know it, eating seems like a daunting and unappealing task. Foods you once considered treats, like ice cream or french fries, are no longer tempting. Obviously, not eating contributes to other symptoms, like low energy and an inability to concentrate on work. If you have lost your appetite in conjunction with other symptoms, your depression is probably getting worse.

How do I know if I meet the criteria for a major depressive episode?

If you are having a major depressive episode, the most pervasive symptom will be feelings of:

- sadness
- flat or muted mood
- hopelessness
- helplessness
- irritability
- simply being "down in the dumps"

An alteration in mood, with a two-week minimum duration, is what you and your doctor should look for when tracking symptoms. In children and adolescents, mood may be more irritable than sad. Sometimes a person may deny these symptoms at first. A clinician can sometimes elicit the feelings by pointing out, for example, that the patient looks like she is about to cry. If you are having a hard time describing your feelings, facial expressions and general demeanor are good indicators of your depressed mood.

To meet the criteria of a major depressive episode, you must have a majority of the following symptoms (*DSM-IV* requires five out of nine):

1. *Anhedonia, or a loss of interest or pleasure in daily activities:* You may have no interest in work or hobbies, not caring anymore if you meet a deadline or win a tennis game. Enjoyment in activities that once seemed pleasurable is gone. For some people, sexual desire and interest also decreases dramatically.

2. *Significant weight fluctuation—losing or gaining 5 percent of your body weight in a month:* Your appetite is reduced to an abnormal level and eating seems like a big chore. Many people feel as if they have to force themselves to eat. Others find they crave specific foods (e.g., sweets and carbohydrates) and gain a significant amount of weight in a short period of time. Children who are depressed may fail to meet expected weight gains, which should alert parents and doctors to a possible problem.

3. *Insomnia or hypersomnia nearly every night:* Initially, you may experience *mild insomnia* (primary) and have difficulty falling asleep. Typically, people have *middle insomnia* (secondary), where they wake up during the night and have difficulty falling back to sleep, or *terminal insomnia* (tertiary), where a person wakes up too early and is unable to return to sleep. Less frequently, people suffer from hypersomnia, or "oversleeping," either in the morning or during the day.

Often, people seek treatment for sleep disturbances only to then discover other symptoms of depression.

4. *Psychomotor changes nearly every day:* Your body movement can indicate whether you are in psychological distress. You may find you are agitated, which can include:

- an inability to sit still
- pacing
- hand wringing
- pulling or rubbing skin, clothing, or other objects

Other psychomotor changes you may experience involve retardation:

- slowed speech, thinking, and body movements
- increased pauses before answering
- decreased volume in speech
- change in inflection, amount, and variety of speech
- muteness

Depression-related psychomotor changes are almost always severe enough for others to notice.

5. *Fatigue or loss of energy nearly every day.* You may feel tired without really having done much. Small tasks seem like they require an enormous amount of energy. It may take you much longer to perform simple daily routines like washing and dressing.

6. *Feelings of worthlessness or excessive guilt nearly every day:* You may view past accomplishments in a negative light and ruminate over minor failings. Guilty feelings about events over which you have no control become obsessive and overblown.

7. *Impaired ability to think or concentrate nearly every day:* Loss of concentration, memory difficulties, and

distractibility are all common symptoms of depression. You may discover a decrease in intellectual and academic functioning.

8. *Indecisiveness nearly every day:* If you were once able to make decisions, both major and minor, with little trouble, you may find yourself now ruminating over trivial matters. Deciding which shoes to wear or what to eat for breakfast may become too monumental a task to accomplish.

9. *Recurrent thoughts of death, suicidal ideation, and suicide plan:* Your symptoms may escalate to such a level that you begin to contemplate suicide. You begin to think that you would be better off dead than to feel so much pain and cause others so much suffering. The severity of these suicidal impulses can range from fleeting, one- to two-minute thoughts, to recurrent ones (once or twice a week). Some people begin making a plan, acquire materials (a gun or rope), and compose a suicide note. Family members and friends are encouraged to report *any* discussions of suicide to a patient's doctor or contact a mental health professional immediately.

How do I know if I have bipolar disorder and not just a major depressive disorder?

As we discussed in chapter 1, there is little distinction between a major depressive episode and a bipolar depressive episode. The only indication of difference is a past history of a hypomanic or manic episode. Gerald had seen his internist several times over a three-month period, complaining of chest and stomach pains, insomnia, and loss of appetite. Additionally, he reported feeling sad and uninterested in his work and hobbies. Like most depression sufferers, Gerald felt worse in the morning than he did at night. After doing a complete physical evaluation and blood workup, Gerald's internist concluded that he might be suffering from depression. The psychiatrist initially diagnosed depression. However, after questioning Gerald further, the doctor learned of his mood swings and a manic episode four years earlier. The doctor then changed the diagnosis to bipolar disorder.

If a patient fails to report a prior hypomanic or manic episode, it is very difficult for a doctor to make a proper diagnosis. Even if the doctor does not think the patient will answer accurately, it is his clinical responsibility to ask about mood swings and prior episodes. If the patient is in a hypomanic or manic state, he is probably unaware of his condition. If the patient is depressed, he may not want to talk about it. The clinician wants to avoid diagnosing a major depressive disorder when bipolar disorder is the true illness. The danger lies in mistreating patients with antidepressants that could trigger a hypomanic or manic episode.

What are the symptoms of a hypomanic episode?

Like other bipolar episodes, a hypomanic state prevails for a distinct period of time, lasting at least four days. During this time, a person must exhibit at least three symptoms from a list of criteria for the behavior to constitute a hypomanic episode. The most pervasive and indicative symptom is an unusually elevated or irritable mood. Additionally, a person's self-esteem may be inappropriately high and she may be prone to grandiose behavior.

Loretta, a sixty-one-year-old librarian with a long history of bipolar disorder, was recently able to detect the onset of a hypomanic episode. Generally a taciturn and reserved person, she became elated and enthusiastic about writing poetry and began showing it to library patrons. Noting this odd behavior in herself, and having experience with hypomania, Loretta called her psychiatrist to report the episode. However, this kind of self-awareness is very rare in people who have never had a hypomanic episode.

You may be experiencing a hypomanic episode if you exhibit any of the following symptoms in conjunction with an abnormally expansive mood:

1. *Inflated self-esteem and grandiosity:* You may suddenly feel capable of achieving feats that in the past seemed impossible. Joanne, a graphic designer, believed that she could handle the work of three of her colleagues and do a better job. When Joanne's boss asked her why she wanted to take on the extra work, Joanne replied, "Because I'm the only one who really knows what the client wants."

2. *Increased activity or physical restlessness:* You may normally run two miles a couple days a week to keep in shape and suddenly decide that you want to start training for a marathon. You begin running six miles a day, hire a personal trainer, and cannot seem to sit still at work or at home. You have a need to always be moving around.

3. *Increased talkativeness:* You feel as if you cannot get the words out fast enough and that other people are talking too slowly. Increasing the volume and speed of your speech seems to be one way to get your point across faster and more clearly. To others you soon seem to be ranting incoherently and appear out of control.

4. *Difficulty concentrating and distractibility:* You begin several projects at home, cleaning out the basement, sorting old books, and writing a play. You cannot concentrate on any of the projects for long before something else catches your attention and you are distracted. Anne found that she had lots of energy at work, but "I couldn't keep my mind on one idea for very long and kept jumping from project to project."

5. *Decreased need for sleep:* Because your mind is racing and it feels like there are not enough hours in the day to get everything done, you sleep less and less. Unfortunately, the lack of sleep can add to your overall sense of agitation and irritability. As the hypomanic episode worsens, the need for sleep can disappear altogether.

6. *Increased sexual energy:* Your once-healthy but not excessive libido can escalate into a desire for sex all the time. You may harass your partner for more sexual

activity than he or she wants, or you may choose multiple partners and increase your chances of both physical and emotional harm.

7. *Impaired behavior and judgment:* Unable to decide which of five pairs of shoes to purchase, you buy all of them. Your inability to temper your spending may lead to excessive credit card use and large cash withdrawals from your bank account. Other types of irresponsible behavior and impaired judgment include speeding or driving while intoxicated and engaging in dangerous physical activities, like skydiving.

8. *Increased sociability and overfamiliarity:* You decide that staying out late every night and getting to know all your colleagues at work is essential to a healthy social life. You want to learn about people's personal lives and expound upon yours even if they are clearly uncomfortable. Setting social boundaries is almost impossible for someone in the throes of a hypomanic episode.

Do clinicians use any kind of scale to measure levels of hypomania and mania?

Yes. In fact, all medical practitioners use a scale from 1 to 4 to measure the severity of any illness. If a person meets the criteria for a manic episode, the symptoms are charted along a gradation:

- 1+ = hypomania (mild)
- 2+ = mania (moderate)
- 3+ = mania (severe without psychotic features)
- 4+ = mania (severe with psychotic features)

Clinicians base the severity of the episode on the number of symptoms, the severity of the symptoms, the degree of functional disability, and the need for hospitalization. It is hoped that a mental health professional will intercede before the patient reaches stage 4.

What is a typical day like for someone in a hypomanic state?

The person has slept little the previous night, then he is up early and raring to go after only a few hours of rest. Piles of clothes lie unattended on the floor where they have been unceremoniously dumped for days. His desk is littered with plans outlining how he is going to produce a Hollywood hit. He showers, singing at top volume along with the music blaring from his radio. Dressing is an exciting task, because he's going to wear one of the new suits he bought last week with his newly approved credit card.

He feels energetic, full of life, and almost weightless as he briskly walks through the kitchen and out the front door. There is no need for breakfast, as he has not really been hungry for days and only nibbles snacks here and there. Strapped into his car, he pulls away from the curb without really looking behind him and cuts off a delivery van. The speed limit signs mean little to him, and he just makes several yellow lights turning to red. On the way to the video store where he works, he stops to buy many trade and national movie magazines so he can develop his movie during the day.

Once at the store, he asks all his co-workers to meet him in the coffee room so he can discuss his project. The co-workers have other things to do and try to brush him off. Not getting the attention that he feels he deserves, he becomes irritable and impatient.

Throughout the day he tries to engage customers, but they too sense his odd urgency and are wary of him. After work he heads for a singles bar, hoping to meet someone who will come home with him and spend the night. Drinking heavily and dancing excessively, he eventually tires himself out and goes home alone.

Each person experiences his very own version of hypomania. The episodes follow a unique course depending on many factors, including environmental stimulation and an individual's personality. People can have calm moments in the midst of their hyperactivity, but it is often hard for them to voluntarily slow down once they are reeling.

How do I know if a hypomanic episode is turning into mania?

If you are in the midst of a hypomanic episode, it is nearly impossible for you to step back and assess your state. Hypomania tends to begin suddenly, with rapidly escalating symptoms. The episodes generally last for weeks to months and may be preceded or followed by a major depressive episode. Usually, hypomanic episodes have a more abrupt onset and are shorter in length than major depressive ones. While they are not definitive, some studies suggest that 5 to 15 percent of hypomanic individuals will eventually develop mania.

One hopes that as your hypomania worsens, family, friends, and co-workers will discern your abnormal behavior and take action. When hypomania develops into the heightened frenzy of mania, there can be several problems. You are more of a danger to yourself and others when you are manic. You are also harder to treat and stabilize. Many people having a manic episode end up in the hospital, where medical professionals stabilize their condition with medication. If you know there is a history in your family of bipolar disorder, acquaint yourself with the symptoms of hypomania. Manic symptoms typically appear suddenly and escalate in a matter of days.

How do you know if someone is having a manic episode?

The symptoms of mania are similar in many ways to those of hypomania. The abnormal mood must last at least one week to meet the criteria for mania. The period of time may be less if the person is hospitalized during the initial onset. There are a few distinguishing features that set the two states apart. Most notably, if you are manic, there is no question to observers that all the symptoms are definitely at an abnormal level. Moving along the continuum from 1 to 4, instead of just being overly talkative, you cannot get the words out fast enough and take no time for responses from others. Some manic individuals describe that their experience is like watching two or three television shows at once.

The symptoms for mania include the following:

1. Mood is continuously elevated, expansive, or irritable

2. Excessively increased activity and physical restlessness

3. Pressured speech that is loud, rapid, and difficult to interpret. You may talk for hours on end, nonstop.

4. Flight of ideas, where thoughts race and ideas pour out at an uncontrollable rate

5. An even more decreased need for sleep than what is characteristic of hypomania

6. Inflated self-esteem and grandiosity

7. Constantly changing plans and distractibility

8. Reckless and risky behavior, including spending sprees and dangerous driving

9. Marked sexual energy and sexual indiscretions with potentially harmful and painful consequences

10. Delusions or hallucinations

11. If psychotic, you may physically assault others and have suicidal tendencies

12. Marked inability to function in social and occupational settings

If you become psychotic, your perception of reality is grossly distorted and your thinking and behavior are extremely disorganized. The psychosis often manifests with delusions and at times hallucinations. Delusions are much more common in mania with psychotic features than are hallucinations.

Manic and depressive symptoms differ in several ways. Depressive symptoms appear in nearly all psychiatric disorders, whereas manic symptoms are more specific, distinctive, and apparent. However, a wide range of substances and medical conditions can cause manic symptoms. For example, steroids such as prednisone in high doses can precipitate a manic episode in some patients. Viral encephalitis, an infection of the brain, can also induce mania.

What is the difference between a delusion and a hallucination?

Delusions and hallucinations are some of the most frightening aspects of bipolar disorder. Patients who become delusional are obsessed and preoccupied with religious, financial, sexual, and persecutory ideas that may lead to complicated false beliefs. If a patient believes that aliens are injecting him with poison, he is having a delusion and may be quite dangerous. He is no longer in a reasonable state, and as his psychosis escalates, he may lash out at others or harm himself.

A hallucination, on the other hand, is a false perception. These are most commonly auditory, where the patient hears voices that are not there. However, they may also affect any of the senses (e.g., visual), but this is very rare. A person experiencing hallucinations is apt to do whatever the voices in his head tell him, and he can be quite dangerous. You should always contact a mental health professional or the police if you know someone is having hallucinations.

Most manic patients are not fully delusional, and many do not have hallucinations. If they become either delusional or have hallucinations, their diagnosis then changes to manic with psychotic features.

Jason, a thirty-one-year-old construction worker, believed that God was directly beaming him messages, a grandiose delusion. His doctor had hospitalized Jason for previous manic episodes, and he had responded well to lithium as a mood stabilizer. Once out of the hospital, however, Jason refused to take his lithium and his delusions set in again. In a subsequent episode, he beat his wife badly and his doctor readmitted him to the hospital. Believing that God was the only one who could truly treat him, Jason again stopped taking his lithium even after his wife had left him.

Is it difficult to treat a person with mania?

It is exceedingly difficult to treat someone in a manic condition. Manic individuals generally do not observe their behavior well and can experience an overwhelming sense of pleasure. People often travel to cities far from their home, neglecting to tell family members and friends where they have gone. They can change their clothes, hairstyles, and entire physical appearance, making it hard for relatives and law enforcers to identify them. When a manic person becomes hostile and paranoid, he can lash out at friends, loved ones, or complete strangers. Until the individual is stabilized on medication, reasoning with him is nearly impossible.

Can moods change quickly when someone is manic?

Yes. Most people in a manic state have an elevated mood, but irritability or paranoia can appear with little warning. People become irritable especially when they perceive that others are thwarting their grandiose plans. Clinicians often observe this lability of mood in manic patients. At the onset of mania, a person's mood tends to be euphoric. As the episode progresses, the euphoria often changes to irritability. A patient's mood can also be at one moment euphoric and the next belligerent. If a person shows signs of irritability, their speech can easily switch from expansive optimism to hostile anger. People who are manic tend to be very unpredictable and should not be directly challenged.

Is mania apparent in adolescents?

Bipolar disorder in adolescents tends to be misdiagnosed by clinicians, because it is difficult to distinguish between an antisocial personality disorder or schizophrenia and mania. Teenagers are known to have sudden mood swings, often precipitated by alcohol and substance abuse. Symptoms of mania in adolescents include the following:

- substance abuse
- suicide attempts
- academic problems
- philosophical brooding
- obsessive-compulsive disorder symptoms
- multiple somatic complaints or problems with their bodies
- marked irritability that can result in physical fighting
- antisocial behavior

All of these symptoms can be part of normal adolescent behavior. However, if the symptoms become severe, include psychotic features, and persist for weeks, clinicians should not rule out bipolar disorder as a possibility.

When do people typically have their first manic episode?

Most people first experience mania in their early twenties. Others have an initial onset of mania during adolescence, while some people have it past the age of fifty. Losing a loved one, graduating from school, or other life stressors can precipitate a manic episode. The episodes frequently last anywhere from a couple of weeks to a few months. Generally, manic periods tend to be briefer and end more abruptly than major depressive episodes. However, a major depressive episode often precedes or comes directly after a manic episode, with no time in between the two states. This means that a sufferer has no period of euthymia in which to recover from the effects of both a clinical depression and a manic episode.

How do I know if I have had a mixed episode?

Knowing whether or not you have had a mixed episode can be rather difficult. It requires that you monitor your mood changes over a short period of time. Ideally, a relative or close friend will track your moods and report to your doctor what they noticed. Having a mixed episode means that you meet the criteria for both a manic and a major depressive episode nearly every day during a period of at least one week. You will experience rapidly fluctuating moods, going from ecstasy to misery and back, accompanied by symptoms of mania and depression. Symptoms often include the following:

- agitation
- insomnia
- appetite dysregulation
- psychotic features
- suicidal imaginings

Fortunately, since most individuals who experience a mixed episode are more depressed than manic, they are more likely to seek help. People who are manic often tend to believe they do not need any attention or treatment whatsoever.

Barbara, a thirty-eight-year-old housewife, was diagnosed with bipolar disorder at age twenty-two and had suffered through several mixed episodes. She had kept a careful chart of her mood cycles with the help of family and friends, which helped her doctor determine the course of the disorder. He could see that Barbara's moods alternated from elation to self-deprecation and irritability, with periods of insomnia and too much sleep during brief periods of time. Barbara reported to her doctor that she had used poor judgment in investing her and her husband's retirement money in risky and uncertain stock funds. She now regretted her actions and felt ashamed and guilty. It was clear to her psychiatrist that Barbara exhibited an amalgam of both major depressive, hypomanic, and manic symptoms.

Why do clinicians find it so difficult to diagnose a patient having a mixed episode?

True mixed episodes impair an individual's ability to interact with others and to function at work, and often require hospitalization. Clinicians have to make sure that you are not presenting symptoms for mania and depression due to any extenuating circumstances. Antidepressant medication, phototherapy (an intense amount of light exposure, often used to treat seasonal affect disorder), or a substance-abuse problem can all cause you to swing from depression to mania. Additionally, general medical conditions, like hyperthyroidism or multiple sclerosis, can also induce what appears to be a mixed mood disturbance. Clinicians who conclude that you have symptoms caused by conditions other than a mixed episode do not count the disturbance toward a diagnosis of bipolar disorder. Mental health professionals can determine whether a person is truly experiencing a mixed episode only by obtaining a comprehensive history and by conducting a thorough physical and psychological examination. The exam must also include a family history of any mental illness.

What is the difference between attention deficit hyperactivity disorder (ADHD) and a mixed mood episode in children?

Both a mixed episode and attention deficit hyperactivity disorder (ADHD) are marked by:

- excessive activity
- impulsive behavior
- poor judgment
- denial of problems

The two conditions differ in that ADHD has a characteristic early onset, generally before age seven. ADHD is also chronic rather than episodic, and lacks clear termination of symptoms. Additionally, people with ADHD lack an abnormally expansive or elevated mood and do not exhibit psychotic features. Children with ADHD often show symptoms of depression, like low self-esteem, and become frustrated easily. However, if a patient meets the criteria for ADHD *and* a mood disorder, including a mixed episode, then clinicians may diagnose them with both afflictions.

Are mixed episodes more common in any one age or gender group?

Researchers have found that mixed episodes appear to occur more frequently in younger people and those over age fifty who have bipolar disorder. Preliminary reports also show that men seem to have more mixed mood disturbances than women, but these findings are preliminary.

What is rapid cycling?

Rapid cycling is not an episode per se, but an indicator of how many mood changes a person has had in a certain amount of time. There is no difference between episodes that occur in a rapid cycling pattern and those that do not, except that you simply have them more frequently. Essentially, in order to qualify as a rapid cycler, you must have had four or more mood episodes during one twelve-month period. The episodes must meet the symptom and duration criteria for:

• major depressive
• manic
• hypomanic
• mixed

Your fluctuating episodes must be demarcated by either a full or partial remission of symptoms for at least two months, or they must suddenly switch to the opposite pole (e.g., major depressive episode to hypomanic episode). Clinicians consider manic, hypomanic, and mixed episodes on one pole and depression on the other. So, for example, if you have a manic episode that is immediately followed by a mixed episode, you do not meet the criteria for rapid cycling. Of course, mood episodes that occur due to substance abuse or a general medical condition do not count toward bipolar rapid cycling. Not everyone who has bipolar disorder experiences rapid cycling, but many do.

What is "ultrarapid" cycling?

If you experience "ultrarapid" cycling patterns (not a *DSM-IV* diagnosis), your episodes of depression and mania alternate only weeks and even days apart. Ultrarapid cycling is very difficult for doctors to treat, and they must be able to distinguish between it and a mixed episode. Patients find dealing with the sudden changes in mood during ultrarapid cycling especially difficult. Coping with so many mood fluctuations during such brief periods of time often requires doctors to use antipsychotics and neuroleptics just to stabilize the patient.

How common is rapid cycling?

Approximately 5 to 15 percent of those with bipolar disorder suffer from rapid cycling. Generally, men and women appear to be afflicted with bipolar disorder in equal numbers. However, women constitute 70 to 90 percent of those with a rapid-cycling pattern. Because women have a higher incidence of depressive cycles, some experts believe that antidepressants may induce rapid cycling. Interestingly, women experience rapid cycling completely independent of their menstrual cycles. The rapid cycling pattern also afflicts women who are both pre- and postmenopausal.

Rapid cycling does not occur at any specific time during the course of bipolar disorder, but it is generally associated only with bipolar I and II. It can disappear just as quickly as it appeared, especially if it is associated with the use of antidepressants. Unfortunately, the more rapid cycling you experience, the worse your long-term prognosis. So far, researchers have not been able to link rapid cycling with a familial pattern of inheritance. Many researchers believe, however, that rapid cycling patterns are probably brought on by external stress factors or drug treatments.

Rita, a housewife in her mid-forties, suffered through a major depressive episode about a year ago, with the attendant feelings of sadness, hopelessness, and lack of interest in daily activities. Being devoutly religious, she prayed every day, waited out the depression, and in five months the mood abated. Two months later, Rita was joyful and elated; she began a grand project of redecorating her home, and she stayed up very late each night reading the Bible. She and her husband interpreted her mood change as a religious experience. Unfortunately, not three months hence, Rita slipped back into her depression. A fellow church member, who was a doctor, examined her and referred her to a psychiatrist. The psychiatrist determined she had bipolar disorder and diagnosed her recent mood patterns as rapid cycling.

Is there any way to decrease the amount of times a person rapidly cycles?

So far it has been very difficult for clinicians to decrease rapid cycling patterns, because they do not know exactly what causes them. When a person is going to begin rapid cycling is also unclear. Experiments are under way, however, with certain medications that might inhibit the number of rapid cycling courses. Clinical experience suggests that mood stabilizers (see chapter 6), such as lithium and Depakote, and experimental medications, such as Tegretol and Lamictal, all act to block the recurrence of both depression and mania.

DIAGNOSIS BIPOLAR DISORDER

What will my doctor look for when diagnosing bipolar disorder?

As you have just read, there are lists of symptoms that your doctor will refer to when determining a diagnosis. Many people visit their internist before they consult a mental health professional because they think something is physically wrong with them. After completing a full physical exam, your doctor will probably ask you some questions about your mental state. If she feels that you might be suffering from a depression or some other condition, she should refer you to a psychiatrist for further investigation.

The psychiatrist will also ask you a number of questions regarding your mental state, many applying directly to symptoms of depression and perhaps hypomania:

- Have you been feeling particularly sad, lonely, or hopeless recently; or have you noticed that you have more energy than normal and do you feel especially confident lately?
- Have your sleep patterns changed?
- Has your appetite increased or decreased?
- Have you felt like going to work or doing extra amounts of work?
- Have you found it hard to concentrate recently, and are you interested in your work and friends?
- Have you had suicidal thoughts?

If you are extremely manic, the doctor may not be able to ask you direct questions, but will need to rely on information from the examination and from family and friends regarding your mood, sleep, appetite, spending, and other symptoms.

The more information you can provide for the psychiatrist, the more accurately and quickly he can determine a diagnosis. He will also be able to surmise certain information just by sitting with you. If you appear sad, avert your eyes, and speak in a low, monotone voice, you are probably depressed. If you wring your hands, keep interrupting the doctor (wondering what you are even doing in his office in the first place), and cannot sit still, then mania is a distinct possibility.

What are cross-sectional issues?

If your psychiatrist believes that you have bipolar disorder, she needs to assess your immediate condition or make a cross-sectional diagnosis. First, she must make sure that you meet all the *DSM-IV* criteria for a manic, hypomanic, depressive, or mixed episode. She will look for:

- psychotic features
- cognitive impairment
- risk of violence to others or to property
- risk of suicide
- financial extravagance
- sexually inappropriate behavior
- substance abuse
- current or most recent episode (e.g., depression or mania)

Additionally, the psychiatrist determines:

- your ability to care for yourself
- your childbearing status or plans
- your support network, including family and friends
- housing situation
- financial resources
- degrees of distress and disability

By paying careful attention to all these factors, your psychiatrist can then recommend a treatment plan that is tailored specifically to you.

How do longitudinal issues differ from cross-sectional ones?

Whereas cross-sectional issues deal with the immediate concerns of an episode, longitudinal ones relate to the long-term nature of the bipolar disorder. Because bipolar disorder is a long-term illness, episodic by nature, and has a variable course, your psychiatrist or mental health team needs to formulate an extended treatment plan for you. Once the immediate crisis of an episode is over, you and your doctors must focus on the future. No two people experience bipolar disorder the same way, so no two plans will be the same. In addition, each will require constant reevaluation and readjustment over time.

Some of the longitudinal issues that your doctor must determine include assessment of prior episodes and evaluation of treatment regarding prior episodes. In other words, she must determine if you have ever had any episodes prior to the current one and how you have responded to treatment in the past.

Will my psychiatrist look for several symptoms appearing all at once when he makes his diagnosis?

Yes. Just because you have predominantly depressive symptoms does not mean that you are not also hypomanic. Eleanor went to see a psychiatrist on her brother's recommendation after she had behaved oddly at a family reunion. Eleanor related that seeing her relatives made her feel sad because she was so much older than most of them, but also smarter because she felt intellectually superior to the majority of them. The psychiatrist noticed that she appeared depressed yet grandiose at the same time. Remember, to meet the diagnostic criteria for bipolar disorder, Eleanor's symptoms had to be outside the normal range of behavior and meet the specific criteria established by the *DSM-IV* for the illness.

What is the difference between the diagnosis for bipolar I and II?

One of the significant differences between bipolar disorder I and II is that bipolar II appears more common in women. Women may also be more prone to having subsequent episodes directly after having a baby. Those with bipolar II have major depressive and hypomanic episodes, but not manic or mixed. If a person meets the criteria for a manic or mixed episode, a clinician will change the diagnosis to bipolar I. Other than that, psychiatrists determine the presence of the two disorders with the same set of symptoms. When making a diagnosis of bipolar II (major depression with hypomania), as with bipolar I, psychiatrists rely on the help of family and friends to assess whether a patient has had a hypomanic episode. If you are in the midst of a depression, it can be difficult to remember a hypomanic episode without the help of those close to you.

Can culture, religion, or ethnicity influence how I communicate my bipolar symptoms?

Yes. Bipolar disorder is color and culture blind, but people often express the illness differently. Depending on our cultural or religious background, we are taught to communicate our beliefs, fears, and criticisms about mental disorders in varying ways. For example, what Hispanics might call "nervousness" Asians may call "fatigue." Some religions frown upon people discussing their feelings, and believers can feel guilty about being depressed. Bipolar disorder may appear to be more common in certain groups simply because those groups do not discourage seeking help for psychological problems.

Will I have to undergo any laboratory tests before a psychiatrist makes a diagnosis?

This depends on a number of factors. If you call a psychiatrist to make an appointment regarding depression, he may decide to run a battery of tests, including blood tests, EKGs (electrocardiograms), and a urinalysis. The psychiatrist does this to rule out any possible physical causes for your symptoms. He also wants to make sure that you will not have any adverse reactions to medications if they are necessary. There is no blood test for bipolar disorder, but a test can help diagnose your overall condition. A general blood test screen includes:

- a complete blood count (CBC), which tests for anemia
- "chem screen" to assess liver and kidney function
- "electrolytes" (part of the chem screen) to measure levels of potassium, sodium, and calcium in your blood.
- "a thyroid profile," usually a thyroid-stimulating hormone (TSH) test, which can detect an underactive or overactive thyroid gland.
- Lyme disease test

Additional tests may include:

- a u/a (urinalysis)
- an EKG to test the condition of your heart
- an MRI or other brain imaging tests

For a further discussion on what tests you may undergo before a diagnosis of depression is reached, please see *If You Think You Have Depression* in the Dell Guides for Mental Health series.

What will my psychiatrist try to determine before making a diagnosis of bipolar disorder?

There are several factors that your psychiatrist must take into account when making a diagnosis of bipolar disorder. It is an unusually difficult disorder to diagnose, because many substances and circumstances other than the illness can make a person depressed or manic.

Most likely, you will first have a complete physical examination by your internist and then a thorough psychological exam by your psychiatrist. The psychiatrist then tries to determine:

- the onset of your mania or depression and attendant symptoms. You or your family are the best presenters of your "history" and can provide your psychiatrist with valuable information.

- if your first episode was or is a manic, hypomanic, depressive, or mixed episode. If you come to a psychiatrist depressed, the doctor must elicit from you whether you have ever had a manic or hypomanic episode before diagnosing bipolar disorder. This is where friends and family are particularly helpful. Men generally have initial manic episodes, whereas women present with depressive ones.

- how long it has been between your episodes. If the time between episodes is becoming shorter and shorter, then the illness is probably worsening.

- what life stressors may have contributed to the onset of the illness. Women often show their first signs of bipolar disorder during a postpartum period. The psychiatrist must take this into account before making a diagnosis. Tell your doctor if your symptoms appeared after you lost a loved one or your job.

- if you have a family history of any hypomania, mania, depression, substance abuse, or depression.

If a member of my family has bipolar disorder, should I tell my psychiatrist?

Absolutely. In fact, he will probably ask anyway. There are strong genetic and hereditary factors that increase the likelihood of whether a person will develop certain mental illnesses. Bipolar disorder is no exception. The closer you are to a relative with the disease, the more likely you are to inherit the genes or tendency for that disease. Ask your parents or other relatives if they know of any mental illness, not just bipolar disorder, in the family. Gather as much history as you can for your psychiatrist. A positive family history for bipolar disorder may increase your chances for the illness even if you have had only major depressive episodes. Once the psychiatrist knows of the family history, she is better able to assess the risk of prescribing antidepressants. She does not want an antidepressant to send you into a hypomanic or manic state.

How will my psychiatrist know if I have any comorbid diseases?

By running a number of tests and trying to eliminate any possibilities other than bipolar disorder. A comorbid disorder is one in which two or more diseases coexist at the same time. If your psychiatrist discovers that you are an alcoholic and you have bipolar disorder, he has to figure out how to treat the two diseases simultaneously. He also has to determine which of your many symptoms are caused by the alcoholism and which by the disorder. Diagnosing and treating a person with comorbid diseases is often a formidable challenge for medical and mental health professionals.

What if another physical or psychological condition is causing my symptoms?

Your complete physical and psychological examination should reveal any other medical conditions you may have. If a doctor discovers that you have anemia or hypothyroidism, that is a likely cause of, or contributor to, your depression. On the contrary, hyperthyroidism, drug intoxication (e.g., steroids, cocaine), or a psychiatric disorder, such as brief reactive psychosis, may be the culprit for your mania. In any case, your doctor will try to determine what the most likely diseases are for the symptoms you are presenting. By making this "differential diagnosis," the doctor is trying to make as short a list as possible of causes for your symptoms. She will then continue to try to eliminate potential choices from the list until she discovers what is truly the problem. It is a bit of trial and error.

How will my psychiatrist decide if I am suicidal or a danger to myself?

If you are depressed, he will ask you about your suicidal imaginings or tendencies. He may ask:

- "Do you want to hurt or maim yourself in any way?"
- "Have you made any plans to kill yourself?"
- "Have you made any prior attempts to kill yourself?"
- "Has anyone in your family ever committed suicide?"
- "Are you unmarried or live alone?"
- "How old are you?" (age can be a major factor in some patients)

It is imperative that your psychiatrist assess the severity of your condition so he can determine the best course of action. The American Psychological Association reports that 75 percent of individuals who do in fact commit suicide have made one or more previous attempts.

When you are hypomanic, you are usually feeling so good that you do not entertain thoughts of suicide. If you have somehow ended up in a psychiatrist's office, he may want to administer medication to make sure that you do not become manic. In a manic state, you are generally beyond reason and your care providers have to assume that you are a danger to yourself and others. Reckless behavior and poor judgment are more likely to harm you than suicide, but mental health professionals never rule out the possibility. However, manic patients who become paranoid or delusional may feel it is safer to kill themselves than be harmed by others. Once your manic symptoms have disappeared and you are more stable, your psychiatrist will probably choose the right moment to broach the difficult subject of suicidal thoughts. Prior to that, close observation in or out of the hospital will protect the patient.

Will my psychiatrist want to talk to my family or spouse?

Every situation is different, and you may or may not want your family involved in your therapy. If you have bipolar disorder, it is generally a very good idea to have your family and spouse be an integral part of your care. This does not mean they will attend every session you have, but at times your psychiatrist will want to talk to them about your moods, behavior, and overall demeanor. Sometimes it is difficult for bipolar patients, especially in a hypomanic or manic state, to assess their own condition. Your psychiatrist should always respect your privacy and not talk to others—even close relatives, as a rule—about your personal issues. Only if she deems it an emergency or vital to your safety or continued treatment should she cross that line. Ideally, she should tell you if she speaks to a family member about your condition.

When children and adolescents are the patients, psychiatrists, psychologists, and other care providers feel that it is beneficial to have parents involved as much as necessary. If a situation is life threatening, parental participation is obligatory. For regular sessions, however, a psychiatrist should never break a child's trust by reporting what goes on in the office to the child's parents.

Does my personality affect my episodes of depression and mania?

Our personalities affect every aspect of our lives, from values to religious beliefs. Mental illnesses are no exception, and the presentation of bipolar disorder is greatly determined by an individual's personality. If you are an obsessive, rigid person who feels shameful and critical about yourself, you may very well deny your illness. You may feel that you are just weak and lazy because you do not want to go to school or work. If you are unhappy, you might reason that it is your own fault.

If you wear a lot of black when you are depressed, you may suddenly decide that you need an abundance of color when you are manic. Or if you are dependent, clingy, and childlike when depressed, you may have a burst of independence during a hypomanic episode. Some personalities literally flip-flop from one pole to the other, causing the person to become a caricature of herself.

If you have a more relaxed, accepting view of yourself, you may cry a lot when depressed and seek help for your lonely feelings of despair. You may also talk more openly with family and friends who offer their support and advice. The same network of loved ones and peers may also be alerted more quickly when you become hypomanic. They may contact your care provider and apprise her of your abnormally elevated mood.

Interestingly, one study found several personality traits associated with bipolar disorder. The patients in the study generally lacked persistence, tried to avoid harmful situations, and were dependent on rewards for motivation.

What if my doctor is not able to determine a diagnosis for my symptoms?

Fortunately, awareness about the impact that mental illness has on an individual's life is increasing. Researchers and mental health professionals are better equipped than ever before to determine the source of a person's problems. However, if you are not happy with your psychiatrist's treatment and diagnosis, you can always seek a second opinion or find a new doctor (see chapter 4).

Understanding the symptoms of bipolar disorder is only one area on which clinicians have trained their focus. Discovering the causes and prognosis of this debilitating illness, a subject we will explore in the next chapter, is another subject of intense study.

Chapter 3

CAUSES OF BIPOLAR DISORDER

What causes or triggers bipolar disorder?

Researchers and doctors still do not know the etiology, or cause, of bipolar disorder. Fortunately, they are narrowing the possibilities and beginning to understand what triggers this debilitating illness. Both manic and depressive episodes are usually induced by a combination of biological and psychosocial factors. Lack of sleep caused by psychosocial stress (e.g., a fight between spouses) may be particularly related to mania. Similarly, if you are biologically predisposed to develop bipolar disorder, the death of your mother may trigger an initial manic or depressive episode. Another person may become manic or depressed after taking antidepressants or abusing chemical substances, including alcohol.

Until recently, many researchers believed that bipolar disorder was part of a long chain of mood disorders that included, among others, cyclothymia and major depressive disorder (unipolar). Formerly, many experts suggested that the disorders differed in expression and severity, but that biologically they shared a common cause. Now most researchers agree that bipolar illness is caused by a series of brain abnormalities different from those of, say, unipolar depression.

In addition to biochemical factors, there are a host of psychological and genetic factors that cause bipolar disorder. Why the brain begins to malfunction at the moment that it does is still a mystery.

How much do experts know about brain function and bipolar disorder?

Researchers are currently focusing on several areas of the brain to learn more about bipolar and other mood disorders. Some of these areas include the hippocampus, a ridge along each lateral ventricle of the brain, and the cerebral cortex. Neurotransmitters, which act as chemical messengers between nerve cells in the brain, control our moods. To function normally, these neurotransmitters, such as serotonin, norepinephrine, and dopamine, must exist in a healthy, homeostatic environment. The quantity and quality of neurotransmitter activity may precipitate a mood episode or predispose someone to bipolar disorder.

Which chemicals are affected in a person with bipolar disorder?

Experts are paying close attention to three specific neurotransmitters, or brain chemicals, related to bipolar and other mood disorders (e.g., major depressive disorder). The primary brain chemicals most commonly associated with bipolar disorder are:

• *Serotonin:* Experts believe that serotonin is principally involved in controlling states of consciousness and moods. Generally, people are more aware of serotonin than other brain chemicals because of the popular selective serotonin reuptake inhibitor (SSRI) medications like Prozac and Paxil that doctors prescribe for depression. We will discuss these medications and others further in chapter 6.

• *Norepinephrine:* Nerve endings and the adrenal glands secrete this brain chemical, which is closely related to adrenaline, the "fight-or-flight" hormone. The sensitivity of norepinephrine to antidepressants in clinical studies offers compelling evidence that the chemical plays a significant role in mood cycles.

• *Dopamine:* According to some studies, dopamine activity is reduced in depression and increased in mania. This chemical messenger in the brain plays many neurological roles. In addition to mood disorders, dopamine imbalances have been linked to Parkinson's disease, schizophrenia, and alcoholism.

How do these neurotransmitters affect the "mood centers" of my brain?

In the past, researchers believed that norepinephrine, serotonin, and dopamine levels in the brain were the only factors that affected mood. Now they theorize that the neurotransmitters play an active role in the functioning of "mood centers." These mood centers, collections of neurons in different areas of the brain, need to work in synchrony for the brain to function normally. If the brain cannot facilitate smooth communication between cells and neurons, it becomes impossible for you to control your moods.

Experts now theorize that bipolar disorder, in particular mania, is related to the "overexcitability" of neurons. To track how neurons communicate with other neurons through neurotransmitters, scientists have developed a numbered messenger system. Externally, neurons exchange information via neurotransmitters ("first messenger system"). These activities then lead to internal changes within the neurons (second messenger system). When someone is manic, their messenger systems (in particular the second messenger system) may be overexcited. Many mood-stabilizing medications (e.g., lithium and Depakote) may effectively work to quiet overexcited second messenger systems.

The research surrounding mood centers and neurotransmitter activity is still in a nascent stage. As experts conduct more neurological tests on patients with mood disorders, they come closer to understanding the overwhelming complexity of the brain and its mechanisms.

What other parts of the brain affect neurotransmitters and mood cycles?

The hypothalamus, which is closely connected to the pituitary gland, controls a number of regulatory functions, including body temperature, blood pressure, heartbeat, and metabolism. Evidence suggests that it organizes motor responses related to pleasure, pain, and other emotions. Patients with mood disorders often have various neuroendocrine, or brain hormone, dysregulations. This suggests that some patients with bipolar disorder may have hormonal imbalances possibly related to abnormal functioning of neurotransmitters.

It is still unclear exactly how hormonal dysfunctions relate directly to bipolar disorder. However, researchers have an interest in three major neuroendocrine systems and how they relate to mood disorders:

• *Adrenal axis:* Researchers have known for some time that the hypersecretion of cortisol correlates strongly with depression. Studies in this area have led to a greater understanding of how the adrenal gland regulates the release of cortisol in people with and without depression.

• *Pituitary axis:* The pituitary axis powerfully influences the function of both the adrenal and thyroid glands. Dysfunction of either gland relates to alteration in mood.

• *Thyroid axis:* A number of people who exhibit symptoms of depression and mania are found to have thyroid disorders. Clinicians now routinely test the thyroid status of patients who exhibit symptoms for mood disorders. However, because many other psychiatric disorders also relate to a malfunctioning thyroid, the usefulness of the test is limited in attempts to diagnose bipolar disorder. Several studies now report that about 10 percent of patients with mood disorders, especially those with bipolar I, test positive for antithyroid antibodies. The research suggests that some people with mood disorders may have an autoimmune disorder.

• *Growth hormone:* Growth hormone, or somatotropin, is necessary for bone and cartilage growth. Several studies show a marked difference in the regulation of growth hormone in depressed patients and those with no mood dysfunction.

What other factors relate to the cause of bipolar and other mood disorders?

• *Sleep abnormalities:* Sleep dysfunctions, whether insomnia, multiple awakenings, lack of sleep, or hypersomnia, are classic symptoms of bipolar disorder. Sleep for normal adults consists of several discrete stages, which can be marked by variations in electroencephalogram (EEG) patterns, eye movements, and muscle tone. Throughout the night, a person alternates between phases of rapid eye movement (REM) and no eye movement. In the first phase of no eye movement, the brain and body are at rest, conserving energy, with muscles relaxed. During REM sleep, when dreaming occurs, the brain is intensely active and several major functions, like respiration, become irregular. Researchers believe that those who suffer from mood disorders may have severe sleep abnormalities, thus disrupting the normal sleep patterns and phases, that exacerbate their conditions.

• *Circadian rhythms:* Fluctuating sleep patterns clearly affect mood and are closely associated with bipolar and other mood disorders. Sleep dysfunctions in depressed and manic patients have led researchers to investigate the circadian rhythms, or internal clocks, of those with mood disorders. A few experimental studies with animals have indicated that antidepressant medications can change a person's internal biological clock. However, the studies so far do not point to abnormal circadian rhythms as a cause of bipolar disorder.

• *Neuroimmune regulation:* Interestingly, researchers report immunological abnormalities in depressed people and in those grieving the loss of a loved one. The depressive episode affects normal functioning of the hormones that regulate the immune system.

What does "kindling" have to do with bipolar disorder?

Imagine you are building a fire and you light several small pieces of wood. Usually, the small pieces of burning kindling will shortly lead to a roaring blaze. The concept of brain kindling is very similar to that of a fire. Many neurologists believe that small electrophysiological impulses in the brain (kindling) create low-level disruptions. These disruptions then lead to over-excitability of neurons that may eventually escalate into full-blown seizures. It is a cumulative process similar to the one that occurs when a person with epilepsy has a seizure.

Researchers now think that the same may be true for bipolar patients, specifically with respect to manic episodes. You may have a series of small, undetectable discharges of electrical activity in areas of the brain controlling mood that may lead to a manic episode.

Based on the theory of kindling in bipolar patients, especially bipolar I sufferers, clinicians have had a great deal of success using anticonvulsant medications as mood stabilizers. These anticonvulsants, which we will discuss further in chapter 6, include Tegretol and Depakote.

What have researchers discovered from performing brain imagings on people with mood disorders?

To date, looking at the brains of those suffering from mood disorders has not shed an enormous amount of light on why these brains are functioning abnormally. Researchers have had the most success with this technique in patients with schizophrenia, consistently showing an increased ventricular size in the brain. In any case, brain-imaging studies have produced some interesting results in people with mood disorders, and current research in this area looks promising:

• Using computed tomography (CT) and magnetic resonance imaging (MRI) to look at the internal structure of the brain, some preliminary reports show that a significant number of bipolar I patients, particularly men, have enlarged cerebral ventricles (the area of the brain that holds fluid). Enlarged ventricles are not as common in those with major depressive disorder as in those with bipolar I. If the patient has major depressive disorder with psychotic features, his cerebral ventricles are almost always enlarged.

• Several reports point toward a decreased cerebral blood flow in those afflicted with mood disorders. Using single photon emission computing tomography (SPECT) or positron emission tomography (PET) scans, clinicians are able to measure blood flow in the brain. A few studies show a decreased amount of blood flow affecting the general area of the cerebral cortex, and particularly the frontal cortical. Continued research in this area will likely tell us more about abnormal brain functioning.

• Researchers are now applying magnetic resonance spectroscopy (MRS) to a variety of mental disorders, including bipolar disorder. MRS is being used to study the brain and plasma concentrations of lithium in bipolar patients. Results from these studies help clinicians determine how much lithium a person needs and how well the medication is working.

• Functional magnetic resonance imaging (fMRI) is a relatively new form of brain imaging. It allows clinicians to actually observe and study brain function, showing both increased and decreased levels of activity in various areas. By virtue of the fact that it is the newest technique, it is also the least understood. However, experts feel it has great potential for discovering what portions of a bipolar patient's brain are being affected by the disorder.

How do neurological conditions affect mood disorders?

There are several centers in the brain that affect mood. Any neurological dysfunction is likely to affect your state of being, and you may present many classic symptoms for a mood disorder. A cerebral vascular accident, more commonly known as a stroke, causes the obstruction of an artery in the brain. If a stroke occurs in the left-anterior region of the brain, the most common area for depression, the likelihood of depressive symptoms is quite high.

The limbic system is sometimes called the emotional center of the brain or the "emotional brain." It handles the emotional and social aspects of such functions as family attachment and falling in love. If someone has a malfunctioning limbic system, which is actually quite rare, she is likely to exhibit depressive symptoms and other abnormal emotions.

If my mother has bipolar disorder, does that mean I will develop it too?

While you may never show signs of bipolar disorder or any other psychological condition, there is a good chance that you might. Data collected by genetic researchers indicates there is a strong hereditary link to bipolar and other mood disorders. The closer the afflicted relative is to you (e.g., your mother or father), the more likely you are to develop the disease yourself. The hereditary factor is corroborated by the fact that nearly 50 percent of all bipolar disorder patients have at least one parent with a mood disorder. If both your parents suffer from bipolar disorder, your chances are between 50 and 75 percent that you will inherit a mood disorder.

Unfortunately, the pattern of inheritance is quite complex and difficult to decipher. No one can truly predict who will begin to show symptoms in a family and if those symptoms will progress into bipolar disorder. What researchers do know is that the disorder often "runs in families."

Do I have a chance of inheriting bipolar disorder if other members of my family suffer a different psychiatric problem?

Generally, families of those with bipolar disorder have members afflicted by other psychiatric problems. These can include substance abuse and major depressive disorder, which many experts feel are all related to bipolar disorder in a family of mental illnesses. Unfortunately, it appears that if children of patients with bipolar disorder develop the disease, they tend to have a more severe version than their parents. One recent study found that if a mother has bipolar disorder, her daughter may be at an especially high risk of inheriting a more severe form of the illness. The same study indicated that if your parents or another family member has major depressive disorder (especially if they developed it at an early age), then you are at a higher risk for bipolar disorder as well.

How strong is the genetic component in transmitting bipolar disorder?

Experts believe that genetics plays a larger role in transmitting bipolar disorder than it does in major depressive disorder. This implies that mania is a stronger genetic factor than depression in bipolar disorder. Researchers think that a few genetic defects must exist to trigger bipolar disorder. Laboratory findings point to significant genetic abnormalities resting on chromosomes 18 and 21. In a recent study, investigators discovered the first genetic defect directly associated with bipolar disorder. The dysfunction occurs on the human serotonin (5-HT) transporter gene (hSERT). Serotonin is a neurotransmitter that affects mood and sleep functioning.

A good portion of bipolar disorder research now

centers on its genetic component. Researchers have homed in on specific genes and gene markers, hoping to link them directly to the illness. Modern molecular biology techniques have helped a great deal, specifically restriction fragment length polymorphisms (RFLPs). However, results from these tests, while promising, often contradict one another. There is still much to learn.

My husband has bipolar disorder. Should we seek any counseling before having children?

Genetic counseling is a very difficult issue to address. Because bipolar disorder may increase in severity when inherited, you may want to talk to a specialist about the risks. Keep in mind, however, that there are no genetic tests yet for bipolar disorder. Genetic counseling can best serve you if you use it for guidance, education, and available treatments.

How do adoption and twin studies relate to bipolar disorder?

Studies of both adopted individuals and twin sets support the premise that bipolar disorder is an inheritable disease. Reports of adoption studies indicate that biology plays a greater role than environment in the development of bipolar disorder. Even if you were raised by other parents, if one of your biological parents has the illness, you are still at a greater risk than the rest of the public. If you are adopted and are showing symptoms of a mood disorder, try to acquire as much information about your biological history as possible. Early intervention can be crucial in limiting the severity of a mood disorder and in its ultimate outcome.

Studies of identical twins have yielded similar proof of bipolar disorder's genetic component. Experts report that if identical twins are raised apart and one of the twins has bipolar disorder, the other twin has about a 65 percent chance of sharing the disease. For fraternal twins, the risk to the healthy twin is somewhere between 5 and 25 percent.

Can time of year play a role in someone's developing bipolar disorder?

Probably. Researchers have not found one single cause for bipolar disorder, but many factors can trigger episodes, including time of year. One study found that men appear to have more episodes during spring, while women are at greater risk during the spring and fall. Interestingly, aggressive behavior for both sexes peaks in spring. A great deal of research points to increased depressive episodes during winter. The common term for seasonally induced depressive episodes is seasonal affective disorder (SAD). Someone suffering from SAD, however, does not necessarily have bipolar disorder. For information about SAD, see *If You Think You Have Seasonal Affective Disorder,* another Dell Mental Health Guide.

Is there a chance that having a baby can trigger bipolar disorder?

Yes. It is not unusual for women who are predisposed to bipolar disorder to exhibit varying degrees of manic and/or depressive symptoms during the postpartum period. After childbirth, your body suffers acute hormonal stress due to wildly fluctuating levels of estrogen and progesterone. Progesterone plummets only a few days after you give birth, followed shortly by estrogen. Both manic and depressive symptoms can signal the possibility of oncoming bipolar disorder, as it did in Joan's case. Within four weeks of delivering her first child, Joan, a thirty-one-year-old former secretary, began to show symptoms of both major depression and mania. At times, she suffered delusions, believing that her baby was possessed by the devil and had special power over her.

Fortunately, postpartum episodes with psychotic features for women with bipolar onset rarely occur, generally only 1 in 500 to 1 in 1,000 deliveries. The risk is higher for women who have had episodes prior to having a baby. If you have had a postpartum episode with one child, the risk for future occurrences with each subsequent delivery is roughly between 30 and 50 percent. A family history of bipolar disorder may also increase a woman's risk of developing the illness during the postpartum period, even if she had never experienced a prior episode.

If you have depressed feelings after your baby is born, do not keep them inside. They are normal emotions, and it helps to discuss them with your spouse, family, or a professional. We can only hope that if you show signs of an emerging manic episode, your spouse and immediate family will alert a medical professional to your symptoms and you will receive treatment promptly. An infant should never be left in the care of a new mother having a manic episode or battling a severe depression with psychotic features.

Is there any particular group that has a higher risk for bipolar disorder?

Possibly. Definitive studies of bipolar patients are challenging, because so many sufferers go undiagnosed or misdiagnosed. Bipolar disorder appears to be about ten to twenty times higher among people involved in the creative arts as opposed to the general population. However, what constitutes creativity makes this complicated. Alcoholics seem to be at a greater risk for the illness as well.

Do life stressors more frequently precede a first episode of a mood disorder than subsequent ones?

Clinicians have long observed that stressful life events generally precede a first, rather than subsequent, bipolar episode. This is true not only for bipolar disorder but also for major depressive disorder. One possible explanation is that the stress of the initial episode is profound enough to have long-lasting effects on brain chemistry. The changes affect, among other things, neurotransmitter functioning and intraneuronal signaling systems. Loss of neurons and reduction in synaptic contacts can alter the brain's ability to communicate messages that alter and control moods. The results of all of this neurological damage is a greater risk for subsequent mood episodes without any external stress.

It is not clear to what extent life events play a role in the onset and timing of depression. The external stressor that is most commonly associated with a person's later development of depression is the loss of a parent before the age of eleven. For an adult, the loss of a spouse generally precipitates the onset of an initial depressive episode.

Everyone in my family is always fighting with each other. Can a stressful family life trigger bipolar disorder?

A dysfunctional family environment is not healthy for anybody's mood, especially somebody genetically inclined toward bipolar disorder. Yet there is still no hard evidence to indicate that family relations cause the onset of a mood disorder. However, a host of theoretical and anecdotal reports illustrate that family dynamics do affect the rate of recovery, the course of treatment, and a person's postrecovery adjustment to bipolar disorder. All of these factors indicate that how a person's family treats him has a great deal to do with his experience of a mood disorder. Clinically, it is very important to assess how a family relates and where the stressors exist, and to evaluate what is best for the patient.

Douglas's father had always told him that he would never amount to much. When Douglas was diagnosed with bipolar disorder, shortly after his parents' divorce, his father told him he was not surprised. "I felt like it was just one more thing my dad could use against me," Douglas revealed. Douglas's psychiatrist spoke to his parents and convinced them that they all needed to come in for at least a few sessions. They had to try to alleviate the anxiety Douglas felt about his family and how they treated him.

What are some common triggers for manic and depressive episodes?

- loneliness, isolation, and low self-esteem
- change in usual sleep pattern (e.g., brought on by change in time zone, work shift, stress—this is especially true for mania)
- protracted pain from a chronic or terminal illness
- loss of a parent, spouse, or child (or the anniversary of the loss)
- divorce or end of a romantic relationship
- problems with marriage or relationship
- involvement in traumatic event (e.g., war, accident, or natural disaster)
- taking care of a chronically ill loved one
- retirement or starting a new job
- surgery, miscarriage, abortion, or childbirth
- friend or loved one's suicide
- physical, emotional, or sexual abuse
- joblessness or homelessness
- life transitions: graduation, marriage, or moving
- substance or alcohol abuse
- change in medication for physical or psychological conditions
- loss or change of psychiatrist or other doctor

How does puberty affect the onset of bipolar disorder?

The onset of puberty and the appearance of bipolar symptoms may be closely related. According to one theory, the brain must be mature enough to fully express the symptoms for both mania and depression. Several studies have found that the symptoms of bipolar disorder manifest as crying and irritability in young children.

In more mature, postpubescent patients, depression and elation are more likely to appear, more or less, as they would in adults. As children mature, their awareness of their mood states also increases, making it easier for them to talk about their conditions if they so choose. It is difficult to diagnose children and adolescents with bipolar disorder, because there are so many variables, like hormones, substance abuse, and lack of an emotional vocabulary.

Psychiatrists can also be reluctant to label a child who is exhibiting obvious symptoms before careful investigation. Naturally, most parents want to know what the problem is and to begin treatment. Some child psychiatrists prefer not to medicate children and consequently choose a diagnosis that does not call for drug therapy. As children mature into adolescence, doctors may become more willing to intervene and begin treatment for bipolar disorder. This is a crucial factor, because early attention to symptoms can dictate the course of the illness over a lifetime.

What are some early-childhood indicators of bipolar disorder?

Researchers and clinicians have established the existence of mania and depression during adolescence. Early-childhood onset, however, remains controversial. There are so many conflicting conditions during childhood (e.g., ADHD, conduct disorder, or schizophrenia) that it becomes nearly impossible to make a definitive diagnosis of bipolar disorder. Emil Kraepelin, a turn-of-the-century pioneer in psychiatry, observed manic symptoms in patients before the age of ten, but later studies have found the onset of true bipolar disorder a near clinical phenomenon. In one study of 898 patients, researchers found only three patients under age ten who showed symptoms of bipolar disorder. The same study also indicated that between the ages of ten and fourteen, the number rose to twenty-four patients (3 percent).

Even though a diagnosis of bipolar disorder is rare in

people under the age of ten, there are some clear signs that indicate the possibility of a child later suffering from the illness. Lability of mood is an early sign, as is aggressiveness in children whose parents have bipolar disorder. Evidence from one study found that a group of high-risk children, some as young as age two, showed abnormally high levels of aggressiveness, lack of empathy for other children, and increased concern about their parents' emotional discomfort. Some of this research indicates that children who are genetically predisposed to develop bipolar disorder learn at a very young age to become caretakers of their ill parents. Children of bipolar parents who are preoccupied with their parents' condition appear to be at a higher risk for the disease. Those who develop friendships and support networks outside the family appear less likely to show symptoms.

What does "thought disorder" have to do with mania?

Thought disorder is a general term that applies to any problems a person may have expressing, conceptualizing, continuing, or abstracting a coherent thought. A manic person's thought and speech patterns tend to keep derailing, much like a train. However, it is possible for a person to have thought disorder without language interference, and vice versa. One definition, offered by Solovay and colleagues (*Archives of General Psychiatry*, January 1987), states that thought disorder "is not intended to denote a unitary dimension or process; rather, it refers to any disruption, deficit, or slippage in various aspects of thinking, such as concentration, attention, reasoning, or abstraction." A useful analogy when trying to comprehend thought disorder is to think of thought content as the lyrics to a song (e.g., delusions) and thought process as the melody (e.g., pressured speech or flight of ideas). Clinicians generally measure thought disorder by assessing the thought, language, and communication abilities of patients.

Not surprisingly, people in a manic state have high

levels of thought disorder (this is also true for schizo-phrenics). Hallucinations and delusions, both of which can be present in mania with psychotic features, repre-sent heightened states of thought disorder. Some pri-mary characteristics of thought disorder in a manic person include pressure of speech (rapid), derailment of ideas (tangents), and loss of goals. A host of researchers argue that manic patients with formal thought disorder may have a more severe form of bipolar disorder than that seen in patients who do not. Supporting this idea is the fact that more manic patients with formal thought disorder have a first-degree relative with bipolar disor-der (or another mood disturbance).

What is an example of someone with thought disorder?

Manic thought disorder can include idiosyncratic and bizarre thinking. The manic person tends to merge ideas, precepts, and images in unusual and incongruous ways. Manic patients often combine disparate thoughts in extravagant ways, sometimes unconsciously incorpo-rating playfulness and humor. Doctors asked Jason, a forty-five-year-old engineer, to describe his job while he was having a severe manic episode. Speaking as though he could not get the words out fast enough, Jason said he worked for IBM, that there were copy machines in his office, that he had ink on his fingers from the ma-chines, that he once studied the Inca Indians, and that he was a fan of the Cleveland Indians. He then began to free-associate and "clang" (a clinical term that describes when a patient begins to rhyme) the words train, rain, pain, etc., until he needed to take a breath. He finished his description by informing the doctors that he had invented a revolutionary new copy machine based on sophisticated mathematics that only he understood. The doctors noted his grandiose and delusional thinking.

Does my personality have anything to do with my de-veloping bipolar disorder?

There are a number of theories about how personality and bipolar disorders intertwine. As we discussed in chapter 2, your personality affects how you express symptoms of mania and depression. Certain features of your personality may predispose you to developing bipolar disorder, but this is usually in conjunction with genetic and biochemical factors. Some patients show cyclothymic traits (frequent mood shifts from despair to jocularity, sleep problems, and shifts in self-esteem), before becoming ill. Other patients have hyperthymic temperaments (overly cheerful, overoptimistic, extroverted, constantly seeking outside stimulation, and meddlesome) prior to bipolar disorder. Both styles may predispose a person to the disease.

Children and adolescents of bipolar parents who exhibit cyclothymia and hyperthymia are more likely to develop bipolar disorder than are others. Follow-up studies of children with personality problems show that early behavior and emotional patterns continue throughout life and intensify over time. Interpersonal difficulties are a primary feature of children and adults who later develop bipolar disorder. Many bipolar adults report that as children they suffered bouts of depression and hypomania long before the onset of their first manic episode.

What is the relationship between personality disorders and bipolar disorder?

The psychiatric community has only recently begun to look at the correlation between bipolar disorder and personality disorders. Some personality types—borderline personality, for example—have a number of symptoms that overlap with bipolar disorder. This can make it difficult for clinicians to differentiate between the two. Interestingly, researchers have found that the coexistence of bipolar disorder and personality dysfunctions is quite low, maybe 4 to 12 percent. However, because information is extremely limited and sample sizes of studies have generally been small, results are far from definitive.

One study found that bipolar patients with personality disorders had more trouble with interpersonal relationships, showed greater amounts of anger, and were more socially isolated than those who did not have a personality dysfunction (McGlashan, *American Psychiatric Association*, 1986). Another study reported an unusually high (23 percent) incidence of bipolar patients suffering from any personality disorder, but the sample size (thirty patients) was again far too small to draw any firm conclusions.

If I'm a creative person, does that mean I'm more likely to develop bipolar disorder?

The list of creative artists who have or have had bipolar disorder is long and impressive. The list of writers and composers, from John Ruskin to Robert Schumann, who suffered from bipolar disorder is especially helpful to investigators, because these artists can express their experiences of mania and depression through images, words, and sounds. Studies of the relationship between creativity and bipolar disorder, unfortunately, have been scarce at best. One small study of writers found that the group had an unusually high rate of affective illness and alcoholism. A full 80 percent met the criteria for a major affective disorder, with 43 percent showing evidence of bipolar disorder (13 percent for bipolar I and 30 percent for bipolar II). Generally, however, researchers need much more data from studies to support their findings.

The same researchers delved a little further and discovered that of those affected, almost all had a family history of a mood disorder. Interestingly, first-degree relatives of the writers had a higher-than-normal incidence of creative activity themselves. These findings may point to a familial link between affective disorders and creativity, but this is only speculation at this point.

One group of researchers at Harvard University administered the Lifetime Creativity Scales to a group of bipolar and cyclothymic patients and their relatives. The Scales assess quality and quantity of creativity in both professional and leisure activities. The group found creativity scores to be significantly higher in first-degree relatives and cyclothymics, with potential bipolar development. Control subjects, those who had no bipolar symptoms, and those with severe bipolar episodes exhibited fewer signs of creativity (Richards et al., *Journal of Abnormal Psychology,* 1988).

On a final note, preliminary research points to an unusually high incidence of outstanding creative abilities (artistic, mathematical, and otherwise) in a sample of children with bipolar disorder.

What is the connection between alcoholism, substance abuse, and bipolar disorder?

Determining the relationship among alcoholism, drug abuse, and affective disorders has been a psychological dilemma for more than two thousand years. Plato refers to alcoholism as a cause for mania, and the Greek physician Soranus assailed those who prescribed alcohol as a treatment for mania. However, in the early part of the twentieth century, Emil Kraepelin declared that alcoholism was not a cause of mania but a result of being in a manic state.

Views differ as to whether chemical abuse, including that of prescribed medications, precedes or follows bipolar episodes. In either case, the reality is that many bipolar sufferers do have substance-abuse problems that can aggravate their conditions and sometimes mask symptoms. Researchers and clinicians must review several factors when determining a patient's condition:

• What is the overall rate of substance abuse in bipolar patients?
• What are the current theories about bipolar disorder and substance abuse?
• What genetic factors exist?

- What phase of the illness is the patient in?
- How does the season influence symptoms and abuse?
- Could the substance abuse mask any bipolar symptoms?
- Is the patient self-medicating?
- What is the person's gender?
- What has caused the most recent episode or onset of symptoms?
- How could substance abuse possibly modify the course of the symptoms and illness (e.g., alcohol can increase both depression and mania)?
- How do we obtain accurate information from someone who is a substance abuser?

It is often difficult for clinicians to determine where the disorder begins and the substance abuse ends, or vice versa. Keeping track of which appeared first is important but not always easy. In addition, clinicians need to monitor the severity of symptoms and pay close attention to family history in order to fully understand the cause of the disorder or the abuse and how they are related.

Overall, alcohol and drug abuse among bipolar patients is several times higher than that in the general population. Some abusers use specific drugs at certain times depending on their condition. For example, one study found that patients reported using more cocaine when they were manic than when they were depressed. Some reports indicate that bipolar sufferers also abuse alcohol more frequently when they are in a hypomanic, manic, or mixed episode, while others show an increase when they are depressed. Still other groups have found that manic patients chronically drink excessive amounts, whereas depressed individuals drink heavily in periodic intervals. Some experts have even found a profound decrease in alcohol consumption during depressive episodes.

Do men and women differ when it comes to bipolar disorder and substance abuse?

Here, as in many areas of bipolar research, there are a great variety of opinions and studies. One study found that 12 percent of bipolar II women drank excessively as opposed to their bipolar I counterparts, none of whom had drinking problems. Among men, 19 percent of bipolar I and 21 percent of bipolar II patients drank in equally excessive amounts. When manic, men are more likely (54 percent to 35 percent) than women to increase their drinking. However, differences in drinking attributable to gender do not appear pronounced during depressive episodes.

Why are standardized measurements for mania and depression important?

Clinicians and researchers need a common language that enables them to both communicate their data and to interpret the findings of others. Experts use measures for mania and depression in order to:

- determine the severity of a patient's illness
- assess and predict how a patient will respond to treatment
- make differential diagnoses
- figure out if subtypes of the illness exist
- determine the incidence of different types of affective states
- understand the course of the illness
- investigate the nature of manic and depressive episodes
- discover symptom patterns
- determine rates of recurrence for the disorder
- correlate information about manic and depressive episodes with other aspects of a person's state (e.g., cognition, personality, and biochemistry)

There are several types of measurements used to gather information, including clinician observer ratings, patient self-ratings, and behavior analyses of speech and writings. Many factors combine to make the clinician's method of collecting data an important factor—namely, a subject's willingness to cooperate, access to family history, sample size of study, and accuracy of information. Doctors rarely use formal scales, such as the Beck Depression Inventory and the Hamilton Rating Scale for Depression, in clinical practice. These are tools more commonly used by researchers.

Despite the fact that a manic patient may not be able to accurately assess his own condition, clinicians should pay close attention to what they are saying. Overall, self-observations, however far-fetched, can still offer a great deal of information about the state of a manic person's mind.

What is the frequency of recurrence for episodes?

Most people with bipolar disorder have frequent recurrence of the illness. In fact, recurrence is one of the most debilitating features of the disease. Even with medication maintenance, most bipolar patients who have had one manic episode go on to have subsequent ones. There is no definitive data on the rate of recurrence, but some patients average as many as twelve episodes in a twenty-five-year period. One study found that patients averaged three episodes and five hospitalizations over a decade.

For those who have infrequent recurrence, major symptoms can still persist in between bouts of full-blown mania and depression. Stressful life events may play a large role in the frequency of recurrence. In one two-year follow-up study of sixty-one bipolar patients, researchers found that individuals with high levels of stress in their lives were nearly 4.5 times more likely to relapse than were their low- to medium-stress counterparts.

Instability of daily social rhythms (e.g., when you get

up, go to work, have dinner) appears to be a major factor in whether a person has recurrent episodes. Patients who regulate their daily activities, or who have spouses or parents who can help them, remain at baseline for longer periods of time. Alterations in your social rhythms—for example, when a baby is born or when you get married—may induce an episode because they represent a disruption in your normal life pattern. Anticipating the stress of a life change and discussing it with your psychiatrist, family, and friends may help diminish both the frequency and severity of oncoming episodes.

What is my prognosis if I've been diagnosed with bipolar disorder?

Even though current treatments are quite effective and are becoming more so each day, most studies conclude that mood disorders have lifelong courses and that patients tend to have recurrent episodes. The prognosis for bipolar I patients is worse than that for patients with major depressive disorder. Up to 50 percent of bipolar patients may experience a second manic episode within two years of their first one. Several of the mood stabilizers improve the prognosis of bipolar disorder, but it is nearly impossible for individuals—much like people with diabetes, for example—to have complete control over their symptoms. However, diabetes is always both recurrent and progressive. Bipolar disorder is recurrent but not necessarily progressive.

Several factors seem to call for a less favorable prognosis, including:

- professional difficulties
- alcohol and substance dependence
- psychotic features
- depressive features
- interepisode depressive features
- gender (prognoses for males are usually worse)

Factors that appear to result in a more positive prognosis include:

- manic episodes of short duration
- advanced age at onset of disorder
- few thoughts of suicide
- few coexisting psychiatric and medical conditions

There is a small number of bipolar I patients, about 7 percent, who do not have recurrent symptoms. Nearly 45 percent have more than one episode, and 40 percent have a chronic disorder. One long-term follow-up study found that:

- 15 percent of all bipolar (I and II) patients were well and functioning
- 45 percent were well but did have multiple relapses
- 30 percent were in partial remission
- 10 percent were chronically ill

It is encouraging that the collective numbers from this study reveal that all but 10 percent of patients experienced some form of remission and 60 percent of the subjects enjoyed periods of wellness.

Bipolar patients with chronic symptoms can show signs of significant social decline and low-level functioning. However, trying to prevent the recurrence of episodes can improve a person's life dramatically. For some patients, taking medication, maintaining a consistent pattern of sleep and wakefulness, and avoiding alcohol and caffeine helps block recurrence. Currently, there is no clinical method available to prevent the *initial* onset of bipolar disorder. If you begin to show symptoms and have a family history of mood disorders, speak to someone as soon as possible. Early intervention can mean the difference between a good and a bad prognosis. The sooner you and your family learn the cause of your symptoms, the sooner you can start to treat the condition.

Are the course and prognosis for bipolar II any different from those for bipolar I?

Bipolar II is a relatively new diagnosis, one characterized by alternating bouts of serious depressions and hypomanic episodes. Experts have really just begun to map out the course and prognosis of this type of mood disorder, and there is little definitive data. However, early findings indicate that if the bipolar II diagnosis remains stable and does not escalate, patients will have the same diagnosis up to five years later. Bipolar II appears to be a chronic illness, similar to bipolar I. Patients and their families need to make long-term treatment and maintenance plans with a mental health professional to promote the greatest amount of stability and normal functioning.

What is the course of bipolar disorder if it goes untreated?

Most important, bipolar patients need mood-stabilizing and maintenance medications to keep their episodes from escalating in frequency and severity. Without medication, the prognosis for a bipolar patient is uncertain and often dangerous. Before bipolar medications existed, Kraepelin studied more than nine hundred institutionalized mood-cycling patients. He observed that some sufferers had depressive episodes that lasted well over a decade. Other pre-lithium reports show that episodes became more frequent with decreasing periods of wellness as the illness worsened. The psychosocial toll on patients, spouses, and parents was profound; all had to cope with longer and more severe periods of depression and mania.

How can I cope with the effects of bipolar disorder on my life?

Everyone who has bipolar disorder has different emotional and medical needs. Developing a support network of mental health professionals, family, and friends is the first step toward coping with an illness that can and often does have devastating effects. In chapter 4, we look at how you can find help—from your intimate circle as well as from other sources, such as national organizations. No one should ever have to face the daunting task of learning to live with bipolar disorder alone.

Chapter 4
HOW TO GET HELP

How important is it for someone with bipolar disorder to seek help?

Very. Frederick K. Goodwin and Kay Redfield Jamison write in the definitive book *Manic-Depressive Illness*, "Untreated manic-depressive illness is, by any measure, gravely serious—complex in its origin, diverse in its expression, unpredictable in its course, severe in its recurrences, and often fatal in its outcome." Bipolar disorder is not an illness that goes away. Without proper treatment, the prognosis worsens and symptoms tend to become more severe. For those who do not seek treatment, eventual suicide is a very real possibility. Additionally, the toll that the illness takes on both your professional and personal life is often profound. If you are given to drug and alcohol abuse, these conditions generally escalate without proper treatment. You are a great risk to yourself and others around you unless your condition is stabilized by mental health professionals.

Many people do cycle in and out of episodes before they seek help. If you are fortunate enough to have an attentive family or spouse, you may receive prompt treatment. Unfortunately, most sufferers do not get immediate help after the initial onset of the illness. It often takes years before a psychiatrist makes a proper diagnosis and develops a treatment plan.

When am I most likely to seek help for my symptoms?

You are more likely to seek support and treatment when you are depressed than when you are manic. Your "observing ego"—the part of your psyche that can take a step back and look at a situation objectively—enables you to assess that you are feeling despondent and sad. You may confess this to your spouse, a parent, or a friend. They in turn may suggest that you make an appointment with a mental health professional. You may also seek help in between episodes, when you are feeling relatively normal, though this is less common.

It is unlikely that you will ask for help and support when you are hypomanic and even less likely when you are manic. You will feel too alive, too "on top" of things to be able to observe your condition. This task falls to your immediate circle of family and friends. Unfortunately, because it is so difficult to get hypomanic and manic patients to comply, they often go untreated until they attempt to harm themselves or others.

Why are so many people embarrassed about seeking help for mental health problems?

There still exists a great amount of stigma associated with mental illness. Most of the misunderstanding stems from a lack of information. Unfortunately, the idea that anyone who seeks help for a mental condition is "crazy" still exists in our society and throughout the world. For many people, especially men, depression and other mental illnesses signify a weak character and an inability to cope.

Families can play a large role in how someone feels about mental health issues. If your parents are embarrassed because you see a therapist and take medication, you will probably feel the same way. Thankfully, the general population's understanding of mood disorders is evolving. Ideally, this growing awareness will generate greater tolerance and openness. Meanwhile, besides your medication and psychotherapy, the most important treatment factors for you are psychiatric supervision, education, and family involvement.

Left untreated, how long will episodes of depression and mania last?

On average, depressive episodes continue for a minimum of six months. Of course, this varies from person to person. If you ignore the need for treatment, the episode can last indefinitely. Episodes of mania, which tend to begin far more abruptly than depressive ones, are generally shorter in length than their depressive counterparts.

Manic states generally begin as hypomania, so it is difficult to pinpoint their length. In the initial or "prodromal" stage, patients may appear wired or elated, but not enough to cause concern. During the second stage, the patient is entering the "active" part of the illness and is becoming increasingly hard to handle. In stage three, the "active" stage of bipolar disorder, the patient may have delusions or hallucinations, appear dysphoric or panicky, and speak nonsensically. It is clear that the patient is behaving abnormally, and family members should take action. Unfortunately, not all patients present such an obvious progression of symptoms. It can be quite challenging to determine exactly how long a person has been manic. Again, each person experiences the disease somewhat differently, but one study found manic patients to be ill for an average of about four weeks. Many studies report that patients who have had one manic episode usually go on to have another, even if they are taking medication.

Experts generally measure the frequency of an episode or cycle length from the onset of one episode to the beginning of the next. Clinicians use the onset of an episode rather than the termination of one because an onset is easier to pinpoint. A patient's medication and therapeutic treatment can also obscure the true length of an episode. Unfortunately, it appears that cycle lengths, the time between episodes, often become shorter after recurrent episodes.

How will I feel during the recovery period from a manic episode?

You and your family will hope that once you are stabilized, your mood will improve. In many cases, however, the recovery period from a manic episode is gradual. You may reexperience several symptoms or cycle into a severe depression, with little or no period of feeling normal. Your insurance, especially if you subscribe to an HMO (health maintenance organization), may cover only one or two weeks of care in a hospital. The hospital will then discharge you before you have fully recovered. You may still be quite hostile and irritable toward family members for committing you in the first place. Typically, the burden of your care falls to your family, who may have to endure your unpredictable moods and occasional abuses.

Sherry believed that a fellow patient in the hospital was going to help her get a theatrical agent. When her mother told her that this was unrealistic, Sherry accused her mother of "always trying to put a damper on her plans." Sherry then went on to deny that she had been ill in the first place and wanted to stop taking her medication. Her parents pleaded with Sherry's psychiatrist to readmit her to the hospital. The psychiatrist encouraged the family to come to Sherry's daily appointments for at least a week to try to help determine a realistic course of action.

As in Sherry's situation, you and your family will need a great deal of support after a manic episode, especially if it is the first one. Everyone experiences an intense period of readjustment, and relationships can be at their most vulnerable. Because it is such a stressful time, support, therapy, and education are essential during this critical period.

Should I look for a psychiatrist who specializes in bipolar disorder?

The psychiatrist you choose should have expertise regarding bipolar disorder, but it does not necessarily have to be the only psychiatric illness she treats. Treating bipolar disorder is a very complicated task. In order for treatment to be effective, your doctor must pay very close attention to drug reactions, dosages, appearance and severity of symptoms, mood fluctuations, and a host of other factors. Your doctor also has to keep up-to-date regarding the most current research, medications, and psychiatric treatments available. If you or your family does not feel that your current doctor is addressing all your needs, you should by all means seek out another.

Local and national support groups, like NDMDA and NAMI, can give you information about referral networks. You may also find out about someone by inquiring within your own circle of friends and acquaintances. Additionally, the American Psychiatric Association publishes a comprehensive physicians directory with biographies of all member doctors and their areas of expertise. The process of finding the right doctor may take some time. However, your persistence will pay off when you begin to receive the best possible treatment for your condition.

Can my family doctor help me at all with bipolar disorder?

Most primary care physicians have some training and skills that relate to mental health disorders. Diagnosing depression is often well within their purview. However, a great deal of research shows that all psychiatric diagnoses, especially bipolar disorder, are underdiagnosed and undertreated by primary care physicians. These doctors can include internists, family practitioners, ob-gyns, and pediatricians. The psychiatric community has had some success educating and encouraging primary care doctors to treat depression. Antidepressants are liberally advertised in medical publications, such as the *Journal of the American Medical Association,* which reaches a good number of physicians. Most internists have no problem prescribing selective serotonin reuptake inhibitors (SSRIs) like Prozac, Paxil, and Zoloft to patients they feel are depressed.

Unfortunately, an internist who is not well apprised of a patient's history may prescribe antidepressants to a bipolar patient and induce a manic episode. It is the primary care physician's responsibility to carefully explore a patient's personal and family history before ever suggesting the patient take antidepressants. Often, even after a careful examination, the internist will still be unable to make a proper diagnosis. Bipolar disorder has too many complicated symptoms to be detected by someone unfamiliar with its course and presentation. If the physician suspects a mood disorder, then it is his responsibility to refer the patient to an expert in the field.

With respect to psychotherapy for a bipolar patient, an internist or family practitioner should really not provide more than basic emotional support. If a patient is suicidal or is abusing alcohol or drugs, the primary care physician must alert a mental health professional immediately.

What exactly is a mental health professional?

Mental health professionals are licensed practitioners who specialize in the diagnosis and treatment of mental illnesses and emotional disorders. Additionally, they are trained to understand human behavior, mental health, and interpersonal relationships. Those within the field primarily include psychiatrists, psychologists, clinical social workers, and psychiatric nurses. Psychiatrists are the only ones of the group who have attended medical school and are licensed medical doctors. Formerly, psychiatrists did not have to know a great deal about pharmacology. Since the discovery that so many mental illnesses have a substantial biochemical component, psychiatrists have had to learn a great deal more about brain chemistry and medications. Today, some psychiatrists, referred to as psychopharmacologists, only prescribe medications and do not offer psychotherapy. They do, however, still provide some psychological support and education regarding the illness.

Currently, some psychologists are allowed to prescribe medications, but not in the case of bipolar disorder. Having completed a doctorate-level course in psychotherapy, most psychologists focus on the psychological rather than chemical aspects of the brain. Most clinical social workers have a master's degree in social work and concentrate on counseling and psychotherapy. Psychiatric nurses are certified nurses with master's degrees in psychiatric nursing. They generally work with psychiatrists or in mental health facilities, treating those with mental illnesses.

Psychologists, clinical social workers, and psychiatric nurses are all capable of helping to stabilize you and, ideally, will ensure the maintenance of your stable condition. They are an excellent source for educating you about the illness, giving feedback about symptoms, and helping you find additional support. However, all people with bipolar disorder need to be under the care of a medical doctor, specifically a psychiatrist, who is familiar with the course and treatment of the disease.

What kind of training do psychiatrists get?

Psychiatrists, as already mentioned, are medical doctors who will always have M.D. after their name. Some psychiatrists have other degrees as well, so they may also have Ph.D. (Doctor of Philosophy), D.O. (Doctor of Osteopathy), or MPH (Master in Public Health) after M.D. Someone who wants to become a psychiatrist must first graduate from a four-year college where they have completed a number of "premed" courses. These courses include biology, chemistry, physics, and organic chemistry. After college, they attend and then graduate from an accredited four-year medical school, where they have several semesters of both academic and clinical training. Medical school provides a general education in medicine. Future psychiatrists must then go on to another four years of residency training in psychiatry.

The first year of residency is geared toward general

psychiatry, pediatrics, internal medicine, and neurology (the brain and nervous system). Psychiatric residents then go on to train in both inpatient and outpatient settings, learn about drug interactions and interventions, and become familiar with the various forms of psychotherapy available. These include family and marital, behavioral, child and adolescent, sexual therapy, psychopharmacology, and electroconvulsive therapy (ECT). The residents spend hours in emergency rooms working with families and patients in crisis. They provide psychiatric counseling and support on both surgical and obstetric wards. For example, if a woman has had a stillborn baby, she is usually in desperate need of support and reassurance that her obstetrician might not be able to provide.

After completing his residency, a psychiatrist must be licensed by the state in which he wants to practice. Some states offer reciprocity, meaning that if a psychiatrist is licensed in one state he can then practice in another without having to retrain. After a residency program, or at any point in his career, a psychiatrist is able to apply for board certification from the American Board of Psychiatry and Neurology. The certification signifies the clinical competence of the psychiatrist but is not mandatory for practice. Psychiatrists gain certification after taking and passing both a daylong written exam and an oral exam. The American Psychiatric Association also bestows fellowships (F.A.P.A.s) on psychiatrists they feel make unique and noteworthy contributions to the field of psychiatry.

What qualities should I look for when deciding whether a psychiatrist is right for me?

Everyone's personality and psychiatric needs are different. You may be referred to a doctor who is an outstanding practitioner with excellent credentials, but you may still not feel comfortable talking to him. In order for your doctor to treat you to the best of his ability, you must trust his decisions and be comfortable seeing

him frequently. A few qualities you may want to look
for when choosing a doctor are:

- empathy
- humanity
- emotional accessibility
- friendliness
- openness
- approachability
- kindness
- punctuality
- availability (e.g., emergencies, weekends, evenings)
- intelligence
- sense of humor

Psychiatrists who treat bipolar patients must be flexible
in both their style and technique. If one method of treatment is not working, they must be willing and able to
try others.

Beyond emotional compatibility with your psychiatrist, it is helpful to know what type of therapy the
doctor promotes. If she believes solely in treating bipolar disorder with medication, you may want to seek
someone who will include more psychotherapy. If the
psychiatrist suggests only psychotherapy, then definitely
look for another practitioner. Clinical experience and
research suggest that you cannot effectively treat bipolar disorder through psychotherapy alone, without
medication.

If you want to know where a psychiatrist trained and
the philosophy of the program, you can either ask her
directly or call your state mental health association. The
American Psychiatric Association's *Biographical Directory* has profiles of all their member psychiatrists, including areas of expertise and interest. For further
information on issues relating to choosing the right
therapist for you, you can refer to *If You Think You*

Have Depression, another book in the Dell Guide for Mental Health series.

Do psychologists and clinical social workers receive the same kind of training?

In some areas yes, and in others no. Some of the training may overlap, as in all areas of mental health, but the two degrees are different. Psychologists spend an average of seven years in graduate school, doing both clinical training and research. They receive either a Ph.D or Psy.D. after completing a course of training in counseling, psychotherapy, and psychological testing. The Psy.D. degree emphasizes greater clinical training and less research. However, even if a psychologist plans to make research the bulk of her career, she must still spend at least one year in a supervised clinical internship. Psychologists must have a license from the state where they want to practice and earn continuing education credits before renewing their license. Most do not prescribe medication, especially not for bipolar disorder patients.

Clinical social workers must also have a license to practice, but their training is usually not as long as a psychologist's. Additionally, they usually do not pursue careers in research. Their job includes the diagnosis and treatment of mental, behavioral, and emotional disorders in both individuals and families. They provide counseling and psychotherapy in a number of settings, including hospitals, schools, prisons, shelters, private offices, mental health clinics, child-welfare organizations, and reproductive centers. Clinical social workers receive either a master's degree or a doctoral degree in social work, with a concentration in psychotherapy and counseling. The course work for the degree combines both academic and clinical aspects and culminates in an examination that is mandatory for licensing.

If I'm unsure about or don't agree with what my doctor recommends, can I seek a second opinion?

If you or your family are unsure about anything, it is wise to seek another doctor's opinion. Many patients do not feel they receive enough information about bipolar disorder from their practitioners. There should be ongoing communication between doctor and patient, yet sadly this is not always the case. Your practitioner has to remain active in your treatment and cannot assume that you understand everything that is happening to you. Often, a doctor will insist on one course of action—for example, one type of medication versus another. In doing so, she may inadvertently create an adversarial relationship with her patient and he may stop taking his medication.

You should always question your doctor about your treatment and ask her to address any ongoing concerns. If your doctor or the psychotherapist treating you discourages second opinions, you should seek them anyway. Do not depend on your primary physician or psychotherapist to provide all the answers. Constantly try to educate yourself and your family about the latest developments in the course and treatment of bipolar disorder.

Will health insurance cover my mental health expenses?

Health insurance companies vary in how much, if any, mental health expenses they will cover. There are continuous efforts in Congress to pass legislation that would force insurers to provide coverage for both mental and physical illnesses. Most plans pay a limited amount, or "cap," per year in mental health costs. Others offer only a certain number of therapy sessions within a calendar year. Currently, most people are insured by some form of health maintenance organization (HMO). If the written literature about your plan does not answer your questions, ask your insurer or employee benefits counselor for a list of the mental health providers included in the plan. Some HMOs allow you to see professionals not on their list, but they may cover only a certain percentage of the fee. If you find a psychiatrist, psychologist, or clinical social worker who you feel is perfect for you but is not on your plan, you can always propose that she join your HMO.

Where can I get a referral to a mental health professional?

The only way to start treatment for bipolar disorder is to begin working with one or many mental health professionals. If you are hospitalized because you are manic, and have somehow never had any previous treatment, the hospital staff will be your first introduction to the mental health world. If you are depressed and want to find help, or are hypomanic and your family is looking for answers, then the following are good places to get referrals:

• Your family physician, internist, gynecologist, or your child's pediatrician can all refer you to a mental health professional. The psychiatrist or psychologist will then determine what the next step should be. This depends on a number of factors, including symptoms and family history.

• If you live near a university medical center, its department of psychiatry should be able and willing to recommend someone for you. The medical school or any hospital it is affiliated with may have a clinic that specializes in mood/affective disorders. Be sure to ask if any of their doctors are particularly familiar with bipolar disorder.

• Any of your local hospitals should have a physician referral service. Even if they do not have an area specifically devoted to mental health, all hospitals work with psychiatrists to some extent. You can also inquire about a particular psychiatrist's training and professional affiliations through the hospital's referral service. Most hospitals also work with psychologists and social workers, but they generally refer patients only to psychiatrists on their own staff.

• Again, physician referral services of private psychiatric hospitals will refer you to staff doctors. However, you have a good chance of finding someone who specializes in mood/affective disorders at a psychiatric hospital. The community outreach department or outpatient services of psychiatric hospitals are also excellent sources for doctors in your area.

• National professional organizations like the American Psychiatric Association and the American Psychological Association have lists of member physicians in your area. A simple phone call, letter, or e-mail is the best way to begin your search. Addresses and telephone numbers for both organizations, and others, appear in Appendix A of this book.

• Some companies contract with employee assistance programs, or EAPs, which were originally designed to help people with substance-abuse problems. Many EAPs now provide counseling to employees who are depressed or have other mental health problems. EAP providers are trained to deal with crisis situations, which is particularly helpful if someone is having a manic episode. Counselors should know when to call for further assistance from a physician or a family member. Intervention by an EAP professional could mean the difference between someone losing his job and staying employed. The service is designed to provide as much confidentiality as possible, but there is always the possibility that co-workers and employers will find out about your condition. Some supervisors urge employees to get help if they notice a significant decline in job performance. There are hundreds of EAP providers across the country, and you can gain access to them through your human resources or personnel department.

• Ideally, every community should have its own mental health clinic. Unfortunately, owing to state and federal cuts in funds for mental health many clinics have been forced to close. If you are not sure that your community has a mental health clinic, call your local health department, state health department, or state department of human services for the nearest one. Community mental health clinics are supported by tax dollars and usually charge clients on a sliding scale based on income.

• Religious institutions are often affiliated with mental health centers. Jewish Family Services and Catholic Family Services are two of the best known that provide services. Most of the counseling and psychotherapy at these centers is provided by clinical social workers, but a good many also employ psychologists and psychiatrists.

• Rabbis, priests, and ministers are usually able to refer you to a mental health center or professional. If you attend a religious institution regularly and the clergy member has known you for a long time, he or she may be able to notice a change in your behavior or mood, either depressed or manic. The clergy member may be able to counsel you, but he or she should realize when the situation demands a more skilled mental health professional.

• Any friends or relatives who have mental illnesses themselves will have a list of providers they feel are caring and competent clinicians. If their doctors are too far away for you to see, one of their psychiatrists can probably refer you to someone closer to home. Using the same therapist seen by a close family member, such as your mother or brother, is generally not a good idea. Most psychiatrists believe that to remain objective and solely focused on an individual's needs, a psychiatrist should treat only one member of a family. This does not preclude having family members take part in the therapy, but you are still the central concern. Some psychiatrists disregard the objectivity and boundary concern and do treat several members of the same family for a host of different problems.

• If you are a student or are affiliated with a university, the staff at the student health services office can refer you to a psychiatrist if necessary. Sometimes the counselors at health services will offer to see you for a period of time before making a referral if you appear depressed. If you are manic, they should get in touch with a doctor and your family as soon as possible.

• People you meet in self-help or patient-support groups will probably have the names of nearby psychiatrists and centers that specialize in mood/affective disorders. They can also tell you whom to avoid and who is particularly helpful. Appendix A of this book provides names and addresses of several reputable groups, or you can call your local hospital's community outreach department.

• For students and their parents, school guidance counselors, psychologists, and social workers are obligated to refer cases that they feel warrant professional medical attention. Again, if the student is manic, the school staff should take immediate steps to ensure the student's safety and good mental health.

• Do not overlook magazines and reference books as referral tools. There are several regional (e.g., *New Jersey Monthly*) and national (e.g., *U.S. News & World Report*) magazines that routinely rate mental health services, facilities, and providers. Several publishers provide annual guides that also assess mental health care, informing readers of the best doctors in their particular region. *How to Find the Best Doctors, Hospitals, and HMOs for You and Your Family,* by John J. Connolly (Castle Connolly Medical, Ltd., New York, 1994) is quite comprehensive. In 1996, the same company published a paperback version that focuses on the New York metropolitan area. Another guide, *The Best Doctors in America 1996–97,* by Steven Naifeh (Woodward/White) should be available at your local library. Most HMOs provide their subscribers with a complete list of all their participating health care professionals and areas of expertise.

• The National Depressive and Manic-Depressive Association offers a list of professionals who specialize in mood/affective disorders. They can be reached by telephone or on the Internet. Information is provided in Appendix A.

Doctors tend to develop reputations, and if two people recommend the same person, there is a good chance that he or she is highly qualified. Even so, if you do not feel comfortable with a mental health professional that comes highly recommended, keep looking. Just because someone has a stunning reputation and impressive credentials does not mean he is the right doctor or therapist for you.

How will I or my family know if my condition is severe enough to warrant medical attention?

If, after reading the previous chapters, you even suspect that you might meet the criteria for bipolar disorder or any other mental illness, then absolutely seek attention. If you are concerned or have questions, you and your family have nothing to lose by consulting a medical professional. This is especially true if you appear to be a danger to yourself or others and if you have a family history of mental illness.

If you or a family member is still unsure, ask yourself these questions:

For Depression

1. Do you have a profound or overwhelming sense of sadness, helplessness, or hopelessness that does not abate no matter how hard you try to shake it?

2. Does working and performing other normal daily functions feel overwhelming and uninteresting?

3. Are you irritable, have you lost sleep, or have you noticed any change in your eating habits?

4. Are you drinking excessively or taking harmful drugs that make you argumentative and aggressive?

5. Have you lost interest in social functions, sexual relationships, and pleasurable activities?

For Mania (this is most useful for families or friends)

1. Does the person appear elated and to have poor judgment?
2. Can you understand what the person is saying, or is he or she speaking too fast and not making any sense?
3. Has he or she slept or eaten in the past few days?
4. Is the person irritable or panicky?
5. Is the person overly aggressive and argumentative to the point of violent behavior?

If you answer yes to most or even some of these questions, seek professional help. Manic individuals will need to be hospitalized and stabilized on medication.

Why is it so important for me to educate myself and my family about bipolar disorder?

The more you know about bipolar disorder, the better you, your family, and your doctors will be able to treat you. Patient education or psychoeducation begins with the process of gathering information that explains the illness, what life stressors contribute to episode recurrence, and the importance of medication compliance. Books, articles, lectures, videotapes, pamphlets, discussion groups, and organizations are all excellent sources of such information. Do not be afraid to ask both relatives and mental health professionals any questions that you feel are relevant. Clinicians have both a legal and clinical obligation to keep patients and their families as informed and as engaged as possible. Information that you and your family receive from your clinician is probably helpful in resolving any lingering confusion or misconceptions about bipolar disorder.

Psychoeducation serves many purposes, including the following:

• Offering you and your family current research studies and data about the causes, course, and treatment of bipolar disorder. Using factual information can be quite helpful when creating a rationale for family involvement. For example, if a study shows that bipolar patients benefit from a low-stress family environment, it helps convince family members of the value of familial support and of improving communication at home.

• Patients and family members often begin putting their newly acquired information to work immediately. When a person is first diagnosed, family members tend to assign blame as an initial reaction. Realizing that a patient is not doing well in school or at work because he is ill, and not "lazy," can offset a great deal of stress.

• Psychoeducation allows families to discuss the very difficult reality that bipolar disorder is a lifelong affliction. When a patient or family member resists this and other truths about the illness, it is a clear sign that there are still unresolved issues and feelings. Family members often deny the truth even after multiple episodes.

• The importance of developing a coherent and cohesive treatment plan. Families must become part of the therapeutic alliance and work toward creating a manageable future for the patient. Ensuring that information about a patient's condition and treatment remains accurate and current can be difficult. Knowing how to investigate further, seeking second opinions, and forming alliances with other families and support groups can be extremely helpful.

What is family-focused psychoeducation treatment (FFT)?

Recent research indicates that treating bipolar patients with medication alone is limited as a single treatment. Most experts believe that treating the illness with both psychosocial therapy and medication is the most sensible approach. Currently, many clinicians feel that family-focused psychoeducation treatment (FFT) is the most beneficial to patients and their families. Researchers have tested FFT in several empirical studies in controlled clinical trials. The clinician's role in FFT is to coordinate, guide, and assist the patient and his or her family through the process.

Outlining the goals and expectations of FFT is a simple way to understand the approach:

What are my goals?

- to reduce tension between me and my family members
- to improve how we communicate as a family
- to help my family to understand and accept my illness
- to help my family create problem-solving methods that are helpful to everyone

What is FFT's format?

- to assess and get to know each member of the family as an individual
- to educate regarding the nature of the illness and treatment, specifically medication
- to improve communication skills
- to help with problem solving
- to figure out ways to solve specific problems

What is expected of the family?

- that they attend sessions when asked and participate
- that they take part in role playing
- that they complete any and all homework assignments from the clinician
- that they cooperate with the treatment
- that they keep an open mind

What will the clinician provide?

- systematic and thoughtful intervention when necessary
- sworn confidentiality for all family members
- a setting where the patient and family feel secure and comfortable
- homework assignments and material
- telephone sessions and consultations when necessary

(*Source:* Miklowitz and Goldstein, *Bipolar Disorder: A Family-Focused Treatment Approach*, New York: Guilford Press, 1997)

How long is the average course of FFT?

Clinicians usually deliver FFT in twenty-one outpatient sessions: twelve weekly, six biweekly, and three monthly. The treatment begins after an acute episode and involves the patient and his or her significant others, which can include parents, spouse, or siblings. Ideally, the initial phase begins when patients are still recovering from the most recent manic or depressive episode.

How else can my psychiatrist help me and my family cope with bipolar disorder?

There are a number of ways your psychiatrist can assist you and your family with the day-to-day management of your illness. Some of these are:

1. Helping you and your family integrate the often painful and disruptive experiences and consequences associated with manic and depressive episodes. For example, many patients feel guilty about their actions during a manic episode and must learn to communicate their feelings to those they believe they have hurt.
2. Trying to get you and your family to accept the

reality of possible future episodes and to learn how to help prevent them.

3. Accepting the fact that you will now probably be dependent on medication to help keep the symptoms of manic and depressive episodes under control.

4. Trying to make demarcations between your personality and your disorder. Helping you learn not to define yourself solely by your illness.

5. Alerting you and your family to the possible life stressors that can trigger future episodes and how to recognize them.

6. Rebuilding damaged family relationships after the destructive effects of episodes.

7. Suggesting other sources of education, information, and support.

How does family stress affect future episodes of mania and depression?

It is not always easy for researchers to determine exactly how a situation or environment affects an illness. Some studies have used the expressed emotion (EE) construct to learn more about how family stress relates to the course of bipolar disorder. EE refers to the emotional attitudes and behaviors of the close relatives of mentally ill individuals. Experts have used the EE format with schizophrenia for many years. Currently there are twenty studies that show that schizophrenic patients who return to high-EE homes (critical, emotionally hostile, and overinvolved relatives) have a greater chance of relapse within one year than do those who go back to low-EE homes.

Two separate studies of bipolar manic or mixed episode patients have found that patients who return to high-EE parents or spouses will probably relapse into mania or depression within a year. Low-EE bipolar patients, like their schizophrenic counterparts, are less likely to relapse as quickly. The obvious point here is that a stressful home life is more likely to precipitate episodes than one where there is emotional support. These studies prove that EE is a useful marker in the short-term course of bipolar disorder.

Family members should not blame themselves if their homes are rated as high EE. Instead, they should view the rating as a useful tool in assessing how to help the family reevaluate and restructure itself. Remember, episodes of bipolar behavior are extremely traumatic to families. They generally need a framework for understanding the whys and hows of episodes. The EE construct and FFT can be instrumental in establishing order where family members see only chaos.

Why do people with bipolar disorder often need assistance getting help?

If you are in the midst of a hypomanic or manic episode, you will probably not recognize your abnormal behavior. When depressed, you may feel that life is hopeless and that you do not have the energy to seek help. In either case, you may also blame your symptoms on something other than a mental illness. Accusing others of trying to stifle your plans or control you is common for hypomanic and manic patients. Depressed patients may feel that their condition relates to a life event, like a divorce, and not feel the need for professional help.

If you are concerned about a relative or friend because their behavior appears abnormal, do not hesitate to get them help as soon as possible. You may face resistance from the patient, but early intervention and persistence could mean the difference in the course of their illness. It may be as easy as encouraging the patient to seek help on her own, or it could entail admitting her to the hospital for emergency treatment.

What if I suspect that someone may try to commit suicide?

Suicide is a very real danger for people with bipolar disorder. You should never take even a mention of suicide lightly. Unless you are a mental health professional you are probably unable to prevent a person from attempting suicide. Even professionals cannot always prevent a determined individual. Do not burden yourself with the responsibility of trying to stop someone from killing himself. If you are not directly related to the person, contact his family, spouse, or doctor. In an emergency, you can always call 911, a rescue squad, or the police. Leaving the person alone even for a short period of time can be dangerous. Keep him occupied until someone familiar with the situation or a crisis team from a mental health facility arrives.

If the person resists your attempts to help, call as many people as you can think of for support. Try to distract the person with hopeful and optimistic conversation. Get him to stop thinking about death if at all possible.

I'm too embarrassed to tell people about my disorder. How can I overcome this?

One of the best ways is to interact with others who have bipolar or other mood disorders. As with many other illnesses, like cancer and diabetes, talking to others in the same or similar situation can be both comforting and inspiring. You will probably encounter other people who have been coping with the disorder for long periods of time. Their "words of wisdom" and advice can mean a great deal more than similar advice even from the doctors who treat you. Jack, who believes he lost both his job and wife because of his illness, found that bipolar disorder had robbed him of his primary goals. Working with a support group and establishing a help network enabled him to establish new goals and better manage his illness.

Whom you choose to tell about your disorder can be a difficult decision. No one wants to be identified or judged based on a medical condition. You are under no obligation to share your news with those who make you feel uncomfortable. Once you understand more about bipolar disorder and have come to terms with the realities of the illness, you may feel more secure about letting others know. However, it is probably wise to tell those individuals you spend a great deal of time with, like your closest friends and colleagues, about your condition. Whomever you include in your support group should know at least the basics about manic and depressive episodes.

Where can I find others who may be suffering from bipolar disorder or other mental health conditions?

Fortunately, the United States has become the land of support groups. Whatever your condition, you can probably find a group of people suffering from the same plight who want to talk about it. Support groups are not only excellent places for gathering information and getting referrals, they can be instrumental in making you feel that you are not alone with your illness. Religious institutions, community mental health centers, and hospital-sponsored patient support groups (see the referral section of this chapter) provide a neutral setting for patients to exchange concerns, ideas, and fears about their illness.

Several national organizations, like the National Depressive and Manic-Depressive Association and the National Alliance for the Mentally Ill, have Internet addresses where they provide supportive and educational information. If you are unable to locate a support group in your area, log on and query these organizations via the Internet. Both sponsor various support groups that are accessible across the country.

What is the Depression/Awareness, Recognition, and Treatment (D/ART) campaign?

The National Institute of Mental Health (NIMH) recently launched D/ART to raise national awareness about both unipolar (depressive) and bipolar (manic-depressive) disorders. With this national educational program, the NIMH hopes to help people:

- recognize the symptoms for all depressive disorders
- obtain an accurate diagnosis for their disorder
- secure effective and state-of-the-art treatment

D/ART also serves to encourage and train mental health care professionals to recognize the signs of bipolar disorder and use the most up-to-date methods for treatment. Additionally, D/ART aims to organize citizens' advocacy groups to further increase awareness and disseminate information to those not familiar with mental illnesses. Working with employers and insurance companies to improve recognition, treatment, and insurance coverage for mood/affective disorders is another of D/ART's major goals.

I know that stress is not healthy for me and can worsen my condition. How can I work to reduce the stress in my life?

The most obvious way is to avoid situations and encounters that are likely to make you feel anxious, depressed, and unsure of yourself. If your parents cannot come to terms with your illness, and seeing them makes you upset, suggest that they come to therapy with you to work things out. If you feel overloaded at work, talk to your boss about decreasing your job responsibilities. Perhaps you can get more time to finish projects. Dennis, a medical-school student with newly diagnosed bipolar disorder, was particularly anxious about not finishing tests in the given amount of time. He talked to one of the school's deans, who told him that he could take as much time as he needed with the exams. In the dean's own words, "If you were in a wheelchair, we'd build ramps. We'll just create our own 'ramps' to make your life at school possible."

Ideally, you will not have to limit the activities that you choose to pursue in life; just keep in mind how important it is not to overtax yourself. If you are concerned, talk to your doctor or family about your plans. In many cases they can help you chart an easier course that will lead to success and stability.

What else can I do besides go to therapy and take my medication to help my illness?

Medication and psychotherapy are central to the treatment of bipolar disorder. However, proper diet, exercise, and an active and healthy lifestyle are also important in keeping your condition stable. The healthier you are, both physically and mentally, the more likely you are to take your medication and go to therapy. Properly managing your illness is the goal of all your treatments, so do not fight them. As hard as it may be, try to accept whatever recovery your illness allows you for the moment. Researchers and experts are working all the time on new and more effective treatments and medications. Have faith in those who are taking care of you and trust them when they tell you that tomorrow brings great promise.

There seems to be so much to learn about psychotherapy. How do I know what is right for me?

There is a great deal to know about psychotherapy, and educating yourself about the different methods and practices is definitely to your benefit. There are several ways to learn more about this important component of your treatment. In chapter 5 we will look at various types of psychotherapy and discuss their pros and cons; you may discover treatment options that you did not realize existed. You should, of course, discuss any questions or concerns with your doctor and family before making any changes in your current treatment plan.

Chapter 5

THE ROLE OF PSYCHOTHERAPY

What role does psychotherapy play in the treatment of bipolar disorder?

Before you can understand the importance of psychotherapeutic treatment for bipolar disorder, you first have to know something about it. When you are engaged in a psychotherapy session, you are taking part in talk therapy or "talking treatment." Using a host of techniques developed over the past century, therapists rely on psychotherapy to alleviate a variety of mental disorders, including depression, anxiety, panic disorders, and obsessive-compulsive behavior. Your therapist generally encourages you to talk about your feelings, symptoms, and any life experiences you may deem significant. You and your therapist engage in a discussion of issues, past and present, that may lead to not only a greater overall sense of well-being but also better medication compliance.

Most people unfamiliar with the therapeutic process assume that a therapist will solve their problems. It is more useful to view your therapist as a facilitator, someone who helps *you* discover answers to your problems. Think of the therapeutic process as a collaboration between two experts: one on mental health (the therapist) and the other (you) on an individual's particular history and experience. Your therapist poses questions and reports observations that may allow you to comprehend yourself, your relationships, and your problems with greater clarity. Psychotherapy is also excellent for discovering negative thinking and behavioral patterns that you might otherwise be unaware of or powerless to change.

The role of psychotherapy for bipolar patients is still being hotly debated in medical circles. Yet most clinicians and experts agree that psychotherapy in conjunction with a carefully monitored medication regimen is the optimal treatment scenario.

Does psychoeducation play an important role in psychotherapy for bipolar patients?

We discussed the importance of psychoeducation in the previous chapter, but the necessity of this therapeutic element when treating bipolar disorder bears repeating here as well. Bipolar patients are best served with therapies that help them to maintain a balanced and stable daily life. A therapist who uses certain techniques, which we will discuss later in this chapter, to teach patients and their families about how to cope with the illness is most beneficial. Anticipating future episodes and learning how to prevent them, a central tenet in psychoeducation, is one way for those with bipolar disorder to learn how to handle their illness psychologically. Psychoeducation is probably the therapy most commonly used by psychiatrists to understand the present and future effects of manic episodes.

Is my psychotherapist the only clinician who can offer me emotional support?

Psychological support is available to you from several sources, not just in your psychotherapy sessions. Everyone from a physician who prescribes your medication to a clinical social worker who runs group therapy sessions can create an emotionally supportive setting. The challenge is to discover where you feel most comfortable discussing the sensitive and often painful experiences you have had or are having with bipolar disorder. Remember, people in your support network also like to hear about the positive aspects of your life, not just the negative ones. Talking to them about fulfilling experiences is a way to make yourself realize that your condition does not always stop you from enjoying life.

Can psychiatrists treat someone having a hypomanic or manic episode in a psychotherapeutic setting?

Not easily. If the patient actually agrees to see her therapist while in the throes of a manic episode, she usually has a difficult time even sitting still. It is a real challenge for the therapist to engage the patient in a conversation relating to her condition. Prior to the possible recurrence of a manic episode, the therapist, patient, and quite often the immediate family construct a plan that will, it is hoped, forestall the onset of another full-blown episode.

Sometimes, when a patient is in the early stages of hypomania, she has enough awareness to get help before the episode escalates. Unfortunately, this is not often the case. Because people feel good when they are hypomanic, they fall heavily into denial to avoid reality. People who have lived with bipolar disorder for several years or decades are more likely to recognize hypomanic symptoms than are those who are having their first or second episode.

It is nearly impossible to treat extremely manic patients psychotherapeutically until doctors have stabilized them with medication. Sometimes, if a therapist or family member sets and enforces clear limits in an unprovocative, consistent, and repetitive manner, the manic person may calm down a bit. Reducing external stimulation, like lowering bright lights or turning down loud music, is another option that may help settle a manic individual.

I'm afraid I might harm myself and others when I'm manic. How can my psychiatrist help me?

A good psychiatrist should know how to anticipate problems and help activate your support team of family and friends. He should also know when to suggest admission to the hospital if he feels you are in acute danger (e.g., suicidal). Once you are stabilized, your psychiatrist can teach you cognitive and behavioral interventions for mania. For example, it is very important for you to have regular sleep and eating patterns. When you are manic, maintaining these patterns is almost impossible. Learning about sleep deprivation and prioritizing activities may prevent you from trying to do everything all at once when you are in the throes of mania. Many psychiatrists have patients write activities down and then prioritize them according to urgency prior to a manic episode.

Your psychiatrist can also help you protect yourself financially during a manic episode. The goal here is to establish some mechanism that prevents you from spending thousands and thousands of dollars during an episode. Written agreements with parents and spouses are a good place to start. You may write, "If I become manic, my husband will take away all my credit cards and my bank card." Other written agreements are "I won't drive my car when I'm manic" and "I won't drink alcohol when I'm manic." Obviously, it is not always possible to prevent a manic person from engaging in some form of destructive behavior. However, there is the chance that if he has had some hand in the process of restricting himself, he may comply more easily.

Quite often, manic patients tend to be very positive. Some therapists use cognitive interventions that get patients to recognize how biased they are toward the positive. The hope is that patients will be able to see their thoughts in a more objective manner.

If I'm taking medication, why do I need to do some form of psychotherapy as well?

It is true that bipolar patients cannot be effectively treated without medication. However, the medications do not work unless people actually take them. The problem is that many people do not, especially when hypomanic or manic. Bipolar disorder can wreak havoc on a person's family, social, and work life. Unfortunately, the disease primarily manifests in behavioral and psychological ways that impede a person's normal day-to-day functioning. Medication alone cannot address all these issues; study after study has found medication treatment most effective in conjunction with some form of psychotherapy.

Additionally, psychotherapy appears to relieve stress-induced episodes. Even though some clinicians believe medication is really all a bipolar sufferer needs, most patients find therapy extremely helpful and supportive. According to a report on bipolar disorder in the Nidus Information Services newsletter, *Well-Connected,* "Therapy focused on improving self-esteem, rebuilding social supports, and making sure the patient complies with medical therapies is essential."

Are there any specific guidelines for psychotherapy with bipolar patients?

There are no formal guidelines per se, because each therapist and patient must plot his or her own course. However, the following list covers some useful points:

1. *Flexibility:* Given the range of types and severity of symptoms associated with bipolar disorder, therapists must be flexible. This is essential because patients with the illness tend to exhibit sudden changes in mood, cognition, and behavior. Issues of control regarding dependency on the therapy and medication compliance inevitably arise. The therapist needs to constantly monitor how therapy is affecting the patient's ability to function and cope.

2. *Therapist style:* The therapist must anticipate, expect, and be comfortable with the patient's wide mood swings and maintain a consistent, interactive, strong, and empathic stance.

3. *In the case of severe bipolar disorder:* Generally, the therapy sessions should focus on the "here and now" and stay away from very emotionally charged experiences (e.g., death of a parent, marital breakup, loss of a job) from the past. Additionally:

- Education and support are very helpful during this time.
- The therapist should educate both the patient and his immediate family as to what they can expect.
- Sessions are often brief but more frequent, since the patient will probably find it difficult to concentrate.
- The therapist must set limits for the patient so she feels safe.
- Both the therapist and immediate family need to be constantly vigilant about the risk of suicide during these critical times.

4. *In the case of less severe bipolar disorder:*

- The therapist needs to assess the patient's personality style, check for problems with self-esteem, concentrate on improving relationships, plan and prepare for future episodes, assess the patient's ability to work, and encourage play and enjoyable activities.
- After the therapist makes a thorough assessment, she can then suggest or employ other forms of psychotherapy, such as psychodynamic or cognitive behavior therapy.

5. Family therapy: One of the therapist's most important functions with bipolar patients is to create a forum for educating, preventing, and assessing how the illness affects family dynamics. Making family members co-caretakers, if possible, can be extremely helpful.

You and your therapist must always work to reduce

the severity and number of stressors in your life. The less stressful you make your life, the more likely you will be to avoid relapses of both manic and depressive episodes. In addition, your ability to function normally will be greater between episodes.

What are some of the issues my therapist and I might address during my sessions?

The issues that you and your therapist discuss during your sessions are very specific to your case. However, there are some general issues that most patients and doctors address and tackle during therapy. Those issues include the following:

1. Coping with the diagnosis of a recurrent but treatable mental illness
2. The emotional consequences of manic and depressive episodes
3. Delays in emotional and psychological development caused by past episodes
4. Dealing with the social stigma of having a mental illness
5. Fears of recurrence and how this may affect current social functioning
6. Interpersonal difficulties relating to marriage, family, child bearing, and parenting
7. Problems at school and work
8. Legal, social, and emotional problems that result from abnormal behavior that may occur during episodes

Most therapists find that using a combination or synthesis of different psychotherapies is effective when dealing with the often painful and sensitive issues that face bipolar patients. We will discuss these therapies later in the chapter.

What is the historical relationship between psychotherapy and the treatment of bipolar disorder?

For centuries, experts assumed that the causes of mood disturbances, including bipolar disorder, were primarily based in biology. Bipolar disorder has never shared the comfortable relationship with psychotherapy that unipolar depressions have had. Physicians, for the most part, were not willing to talk or listen to patients with bipolar disorder about their condition, but used cures that sought to physically adjust the brain. These included mineral baths, bloodletting, herbs, vapors, opiates, warm water, cold water, and physical restraints.

Psychoanalysts like Freud and other pioneers of psychotherapy did not consider mood disorder patients good subjects for psychoanalytic methods. Some practitioners found bipolar patients impatient, envious, exploitative, possessive, and lacking in complexity and subtlety. One psychoanalyst, S. Rado, remarked in 1928 that bipolar patients were continually caught up in a "raging orgy of self-torture." Clinicians tended to lump bipolar patients and schizophrenics together and found them generally lacking in introspection. Bipolar patients also appeared to have an uncanny ability to confound their therapists.

Despite these early beliefs, a strong core of analysts remained committed to treating patients with mood disturbances. Once clinicians began administering lithium to bipolar patients, enthusiasm for including them in serious psychotherapeutic treatment increased tremendously. Conversing with them, quite frankly, became much easier.

Early psychotherapists and psychoanalysts added much to the overall understanding of bipolar disorder, as many kept detailed notes and descriptions of their sessions with patients. Their observations detail what it was like to try to treat bipolar patients before the onset of medication. Their conceptions of the illness have

greatly affected current clinical and ethical considerations in the treatment of bipolar disorder.

How does psychotherapy differ from counseling?

Psychotherapy and counseling share many qualities, but
they also differ in fundamental ways. Those who counsel generally present a series of options to you, trying to
get you to make your own life choices. The burden is on
the counselor to clearly outline how to solve the problem and then let you make your own way. Psychotherapists are more likely to help you recognize negative and
destructive life patterns and help you make decisions to
break those patterns. Counseling can be brief or extended, and it is useful for providing hope, guidelines,
and information. It is also helpful for people who have
a specific problem to solve—for example, a newly married couple who need some guidance in learning how to
communicate with each other.

Psychotherapy generally demands a greater commitment of time and self-exploration than does counseling.
The relationship you develop with your therapist tends
to be more intimate, profound, and longer-lasting than
one you would create with a counselor. Psychotherapy
carries the presumption that there is a great deal of
work you wish to do toward understanding the issues in
your life. There are two primary psychological mechanisms that must work together for psychotherapy to be
successful:

1. *The therapeutic alliance:* This is the conscious,
working relationship you develop and sustain with your
therapist. The alliance is fundamental for learning to
trust your therapist, to identify destructive behavior,
and to work toward a healthy resolution of problems.

2. *Transference:* While working with your therapist,
you unconsciously transfer emotions, thoughts, and reactions toward the significant people in your life onto
your therapist. Your therapist is trained to understand
and cope with how you may treat him during an effec-

tive transference, no matter how positive or negative. In the safe setting of your therapy sessions, working through all the transference feelings is both healthy and cathartic.

The therapeutic alliance and transference can both exist in a counseling session, but usually they are less intense.

If I have bipolar disorder, can I see a psychologist or a clinical social worker rather than a psychiatrist?

No. Bipolar patients need to work with a psychiatrist who is knowledgeable about the complexities of the illness. Many psychologists and social workers certainly know a great deal about bipolar disorder, but they may not be up to date on, for example, the latest drug treatments, the cutting-edge clinical research, and seasonal patterns of the illness. In addition, they are not legally able to prescribe bipolar medication. This does not mean you cannot seek adjunctive forms of support from psychologists, social workers, and the groups that many of them run. It is beneficial to develop a long-term relationship with a psychiatrist who will come to know your moods and patterns over an extended period of time. You and your doctor must track the course of your illness together so you can jointly make modifications in your treatment when necessary.

What is cognitive-behavioral therapy (CBT)?

According to recent research, cognitive-behavioral therapy, or CBT, appears to be an extremely promising adjunctive treatment, with medication, for bipolar disorder. The central aim of CBT is to stop patients from perpetuating negative and distorted beliefs about themselves, their immediate environment, and the future. Experts believe that pessimistic attitudes and low self-esteem perpetuate episodes of both depression and hypomania.

Therapists try to teach problem-solving strategies in

an attempt to lessen relapse rates. Other therapists adopt the technique of stopping patients from "spiraling" downward in a progression of negativity. For example, a patient may begin his session by commenting on how much rain is falling outside. This leads him to state how much rainy days depress him, thus reminding him that nothing in his life makes him happy. He feels worthless and a failure because he cannot hold down a job or meet someone to marry. The therapist guides the patient away from these thoughts and tries to get him to focus on more positive aspects of himself. One way the therapist can activate more positive thinking is to have the patient keep a log of negative thoughts, which he then rewrites into positive ones. For example, instead of "The rain reminds me how miserable I am," the patient might write "The rain is good for plants and flowers, and flowers always cheer me up."

When Aaron T. Beck developed CBT at the University of Pennsylvania in the 1970s, he literally reversed Freudian psychology. Freud maintained that how we feel influences our thinking, whereas CBT purports that how we think determines how we feel. Dr. Noreen Reilly-Harrington of the Massachusetts General Hospital in Boston, developed a twelve-session CBT protocol that she designed to identify cognitive errors associated with depression and mania. Additionally, this design helps to reduce the impact of stress on a patient's life through problem-solving techniques, and challenges distorted beliefs about medication. Dr. Reilly-Harrington also found that patients complied with medications more frequently when she enlisted family members to sign a "treatment contract."

The sad truth is that experts really know very little when it comes to bipolar disorder and psychotherapy. The goals of CBT are to ultimately improve the quality of the bipolar patient's life by giving him tools to reduce symptoms, remain optimistic, and prevent recurrence of episodes.

How does cognitive-behavioral therapy use psychosocial treatments to help patients?

Psychosocial skills acquisition is a central tenet in CBT. Participants are encouraged to connect cognitive errors and associated feelings with abnormal behavior such as sexual indiscretions and excessive spending. The aim of psychosocial treatments is to repair and nurture interpersonal behaviors necessary for patient independence and survival within a community. Patients need to have supportive and socially rewarding relationships in order to feel they are functioning normally within society.

Therapists often use role playing for acquiring necessary social skills. The role-playing method helps to uncover certain behavioral problems that arise during treatment. Social skills training aims to create an environment where patients begin to initiate positive comments, listen empathically, make positive requests for action, express negative feelings in a direct manner, and acknowledge pleasurable events. Patients benefit from both a group setting and individual training when working on these skills.

What are the other types of therapies my psychiatrist might use while treating me?

As stated earlier, most therapists use an amalgam of psychotherapeutic techniques, depending on the needs of their patients. The various disciplines include the following:

- *Interpersonal psychotherapy (IPT):* Developed by Gerald Klerman and Myrna Weissman, and further refined by John Markowitz at Cornell University Medical College, this therapy is based on two basic assumptions:

    1. A patient's current interpersonal problems (the conflicts, distortions, and difficulties they have with others) have their roots in earlier dysfunctional relationships.

2. A person's current interpersonal problems
    play a direct role in precipitating and perpetu-
    ating symptoms.

The treatment focuses on one or two of the patient's
current problems with others to understand past patterns of behavior and moods. In clinical trials, researchers have found that IPT is very helpful in the treatment
of major depressive disorder. The IPT program generally consists of twelve to sixteen weekly sessions, and
goals include reducing symptoms, enhancing self-
esteem, and improving social functioning. Therapists
actively work with patients during sessions, trying to
get them to understand how unhealthy relationships
and reactions to those relationships directly relate to
their symptoms.

• *Behavior psychotherapy:* Behavior therapy is based
on the theory that when a person has maladaptive behavioral patterns, he receives little or no positive feedback. Sometimes he is rejected from his immediate circle
and society in general. However, the person knows how
to get a reaction from those around him only by using
negative behaviors. The derisive attention he receives is,
in his mind, better than nothing. The goal of the therapy is to look at these self-destructive behaviors, learn
how to readjust them, and exchange negative reactions
for positive reinforcement. Therapists also often teach
patients several relaxation techniques to calm moods.

• *Classic psychoanalysis:* Psychoanalysis, developed by
Sigmund Freud (1856–1939), is probably not the best
form of psychotherapy for people with severe mood disorders. The patient lies on a couch, not looking at the
therapist, and speaks of whatever comes to mind
through a "stream of consciousness." The therapist is
not interactive with the patient and therefore cannot
offer many suggestions on how to alter destructive behavior. The patient spends a great deal of time, up to
five sessions per week, examining how the components
of his childhood combined to create his or her personal-

ity. Psychoanalysis is not a good choice of therapy for someone with a mood disorder, unipolar or bipolar, because it does not address the need to modify one's life and comply with medication. Additionally, psychoanalysis tends to require that the patient experience heightened states of anxiety and distress throughout the course of treatment. The technique is better suited for those who want to spend several years investigating their personality structure and perhaps change it significantly. Some of the aims of psychoanalysis include improvements in trust, intimacy, coping mechanisms, grieving capacity, and the ability to experience a wide range of emotions. A skilled practitioner is able to use elements of Freud's theories with her mood disorder patients, but will probably not suggest an ample dose of psychoanalysis.

• *Psychoanalytically oriented therapy:* Sometimes called psychodynamic psychiatry, this form of therapy uses psychoanalytic theory and principles, but patients and therapists are more interactive, usually sitting face-to-face. Brief psychodynamic therapies are useful modalities for exploring the personality of a bipolar patient who is not profoundly depressed or manic.

• *Family therapy:* Many psychiatrists no longer view family therapy as a secondary form of treatment for their bipolar patients. Meeting with family members, spouses, and sometimes close friends of the patient helps to strengthen the patient's emotional and social supports. Involving the family and close friends also serves to reduce stress in the patient's life, which helps prevent the recurrence of episodes. The therapy examines several major facets of a person's family life, including:

1. The bipolar patient's role in the family and how he or she relates to the overall psychological well-being of the entire family

2. Outlining for the family how they can help

maintain and prevent future symptoms and
episodes

3. Family dynamics and how members interact
    with each other

The family has to work hard at encouraging the patient to continue with therapy and medication compliance, especially because of the high risk of suicide in
bipolar patients. The family should never make the patient feel guilty about her condition, because the illness
is in no way her fault. On the other hand, therapists
must caution family members against becoming en-
ablers. Sometimes it is necessary to be firm and strong
when trying to get patients to take their medications.
Family therapy, which has a strong psychoeducational
component with respect to bipolar disorder, also af-
fords parents, spouses, siblings, and children an opportunity to address their own needs. Caring for a mentally
ill relative can take a severe toll on family members that
can lead to their own bouts with anxiety and depression. Therapy helps family members realize that they do
not have to take care of the patient themselves and that
they should take periodic breaks from their familial duties.

• *Group therapy:* According to Irene Patelis-Siotis,
M.D., who is currently a primary investigator in a study
of CBT and bipolar patients, there "is something really
powerful that happens with groups, particularly for
people who have chronic disorders." For example, in a
group setting, participants can practice skills on each
other in a way that is not possible during individual
therapy sessions. Modeling behavior and replicating social situations is an opportunity for bipolar patients to
express their fears, doubts, concerns, and feelings to
others with similar problems in a secure and safe environment. Alleviating the sense of isolation and the fear
of social stigma that bipolar patients live with is another
great benefit of group therapy.

• *Couples therapy:* Not surprisingly, people with bipolar disorder have a high rate of divorce. According to one study, about 50 percent of all spouses report that they would not have gotten married or had children if they had known the other spouse was going to develop a mood disorder. The findings of this and other studies strongly suggest that couples struggling with the ups and downs of bipolar disorder need a place to discuss their relationship. Therapists can offer coping skills for both spouses, trying to make the burden of care rest equally on both the husband's and the wife's shoulders. Often, becoming partners in maintaining a healthy and functioning home life helps alleviate feelings of guilt and resentment on both sides. Bipolar patients and their spouses probably need to work with the patient's psychiatrist unless the doctor recommends a marriage counselor. The couple must realize, however, that their problems generally go beyond a general couples counselor's training.

Are there any other forms of psychotherapy?

Briefly, the other forms include the following:

• *Supportive psychotherapy:* The focus of this therapy is the "here and now." The therapist, generally a psychologist or social worker, offers a great deal of guidance, direction, advice, and support. Supportive psychotherapy can last anywhere from a few weeks to years, depending on the patient's condition, progress, and need.

• *Brief psychotherapy:* There are several models for brief psychotherapy, most notably a shortened version of traditional psychodynamic psychotherapy. Therapists using brief therapies generally try to establish specific goals for patients. For example, a patient may try to understand how his past has led to a current depression. Patients should not take "brief" too literally, as therapy can last much longer than just a few weeks. This therapy is not recommended for bipolar patients, since their treatment plans need to be long-term and not brief.

• *Pluralistic psychotherapy:* For the patient who does not respond well to only one type of psychotherapy, a pluralistic approach can be useful. Most therapists do in fact combine many aspects of all the therapeutic modalities, depending on the needs of the patient. For example, cognitive techniques and psychodynamics can help bipolar patients to see that how they think affects how they feel about a situation. Therapists need to have a firm grasp of all the possible techniques and how they might apply to patients before attempting to decide on an effective treatment. Knowing the benefits and risks of certain therapies with bipolar patients is fundamental.

Where do people go for therapy sessions?

There are many different sites and settings where patients can engage in meaningful and beneficial psychotherapeutic treatment. If you see a psychiatrist or therapist privately, you will probably go to a building where she maintains an office or to an office in her home. Some therapists see patients, either in groups or individually, in community mental health centers and outpatient clinics. Generally, it is up to the care provider to choose the setting where you will have your sessions, but sometimes the patient has a say in the matter. For example, if your therapist wants to include some family members, it may be more convenient to see them at home. However, seeing patients with their families in a neutral environment is usually a better idea.

If you are having an acute bipolar episode and your doctor or family has you hospitalized, then you will probably have at least a few sessions in an inpatient setting. If you stay in the hospital for any period of time after stabilization or are transferred to another care facility (e.g., a partial hospital) outside the hospital, your psychotherapy will continue. Additionally, if you are in a care facility with other patients, you will probably be asked to take part in some form of group therapy.

Ideally, you will act as a partner with your doctor and family in making treatment decisions. If your judgment is so impaired that they feel you are a danger to yourself and others, then your caretakers will have to make decisions without you. When you are in a reasonable state, your psychiatrist and other therapists should make a considerable effort to work to make you and your family understand the reasons for certain treatment recommendations. Long-term relationships with doctors and other caretakers can make these conversations and choices easier.

What if I'm unable to make treatment decisions for myself, including hospitalization?

Every state has different guidelines regarding involuntary commitment to hospitals for mentally ill patients. Many, like New York, require the signatures of two doctors to commit a patient to a hospital against his will. Manic patients appear to be capable of presenting different pictures of themselves to different parties (e.g., doctors, family members, judges), thus making a unanimous decision regarding hospitalization quite difficult. The psychiatrist's duty in such cases is to educate the other parties regarding the nature of mania and the importance of closely monitored treatment.

Patients who may need to be fully or partially hospitalized without their consent include:

- those who are incapable of cooperating with treatment
- those whose judgment is so impaired that they cannot care for themselves
- those who are at risk for suicide or homicide
- those with other psychiatric or medical conditions that may make outpatient treatment unsafe

Discussing treatment settings with your psychiatrist ahead of time is preferable to not knowing your options in the event of an acute episode. Your doctor should always choose the least restrictive environment (e.g., one that limits your personal freedom the least) whenever possible. It may be difficult to face such realities, but ultimately, talking things over will make your treatment experience that much more effective.

How often is unconscious denial a factor in disruption of treatment for bipolar disorder?

Quite often. Every individual responds to her diagnosis and treatment plan in her own way. Some are more willing than others to accept their illness from its onset. Most patients experience a certain amount of unconscious denial, conscious anger, and certainly ambivalence regarding the grave reality that they have a chronic mental illness. Therapists need to work with their bipolar patients over long periods of time. Ideally, once the patient has lived with the condition for a certain amount of time, and seen how noncompliance can ravage her life, she will stop denying reality. With denial out of the way, she can then begin to learn new ways of coping with the illness rather than merely living with it.

What percentage of bipolar patients respond to psychotherapy?

Unfortunately, there is not enough research to say accurately what percentage of bipolar patients respond to psychotherapeutic treatments. Current data does indicate that patients appear to do well when their therapy focuses on changing negative attitudes about themselves and their illnesses to more positive ones. Studies with cognitive behavioral therapy show this form to be more effective than other therapies. In a study of thirty individuals suffering from bipolar disorder, Professor Jan Scott of England found that the cognitive behavioral approach seemed to be acceptable and helpful to about 60 percent of the people in the group. Dr. Irene Patelis-

Siotis, who has studied group cognitive therapy treatment on a number of bipolar subjects, believes that "the ingredients for change are the group treatment and skill acquisition and the ability to cope better and live better with the illness."

Every form of psychotherapy, from supportive to psychoeducational, adds a humane and empathic element that medication treatment alone cannot offer. It would be ideal if all forms of psychotherapy benefited bipolar patients, but this is not always the case. It is just as important for researchers to determine which types of psychotherapies are not useful to bipolar patients as to determine those that are. Some alternative forms, which we will look at in chapter 7, are actually harmful to bipolar patients because they have the potential to induce mania.

How will my therapist know which psychotherapy is best for me?

If you meet the criteria for bipolar disorder, are diagnosed with the illness, and begin psychotherapy, your therapist should take the time to determine which modality is right for you. Psychotherapy, even brief therapy, is not a fast process, but rather one that reveals its benefits over time. As mentioned earlier, your therapist will probably use a combination of techniques, including supportive and cognitive-behavioral therapy, in order to afford you optimal long-term treatment.

Cognitive-behavioral therapy is gaining wide credence as a very effective form of treatment. Following is a composite sketch of a patient with bipolar disorder receiving cognitive-behavioral therapy:

Lawrence, a forty-eight-year-old editor, was recently laid off from work when a large conglomerate bought the magazine for which he worked. Lawrence had been diagnosed with bipolar disorder in his early thirties and had had a number of both depressive and hypomanic episodes since the onset of the illness. He had taken lithium for many years, but his doctor switched him to

Depakote after he complained of lithium-related side effects. Lawrence had been seeing the same psychiatrist for ten years and was very comfortable with his weekly psychotherapy sessions.

After Lawrence lost his job, he assumed that he had been fired because his work was no longer acceptable. Lawrence told his therapist that "I've lost my ability to spot ideas and have no talent for editing. I don't know who would want to hire me now. I think my professional life is over." After determining Lawrence's mood fluctuations, sleeping patterns, and appetite over the past few weeks, his psychiatrist asked Lawrence if he could remember any of the good things his boss had said to him before letting him go. He also asked Lawrence to list all of the awards he had received for his editing over the years and how many colleagues had come to the company party thrown in his honor. Lawrence began to realize that he had made a difference at the magazine and that he was not to blame for his being fired. His psychiatrist urged Lawrence to look at all the other positive aspects of his life: his wife of twenty-five years, his son, and his volunteer work at a local mental health clinic for outpatients. Cognitive-behavioral therapy helped Lawrence to see how his depression-influenced moods distorted his self-image, his thinking patterns, and his feelings about himself. His psychiatrist continued to work with Lawrence, using CBT almost exclusively, until he found a new job and better realized how external changes affect his moods and outlook.

Lawrence's psychiatrist also suggested that he take part in the mood disorder therapy group at the outpatient clinic. There Lawrence would have an opportunity to share with others affected by mood disorders his observations on his recent stressful life event. He could learn coping skills that others had acquired when faced with similar situations and circumstances.

Will my health insurance cover psychotherapy?

Your coverage will depend on what type of plan you have and your official diagnosis. Most insurance companies and HMOs have very limited coverage for psychiatric disorders, placing either annual or lifetime caps on treatment. If you are being treated in a hospital or partial hospital setting after an acute episode, you may have greater coverage. Unfortunately, most people currently pay out-of-pocket for extended psychotherapeutic care. One thing to keep in mind is that individual care is far more expensive than group therapy. Researchers are often looking for subjects on which to test psychotherapeutic techniques, and these are often free. For more information about current studies, try calling local medical schools or hospitals with a psychiatric unit. In addition, national organizations like the National Alliance for the Mentally Ill (see Appendix A) may have information on studies being conducted in your area.

Is it important for my therapist to remember everything I've said during past sessions?

Your therapist should be well-trained in remembering a great deal of what you have discussed during your sessions. However, many therapists use the aid of handwritten notes and occasionally recorded audiotapes (with your permission) to help them keep track of your therapy. After a while, your therapist should be familiar enough with you and your case that he or she needs only a few words or phrases to recall the important issues of your treatment. Therapists see dozens of patients, and it is part of their job to distinguish among them and their problems. For most seasoned and well-trained therapists, memorizing what takes place during a therapy session has become second nature.

How long do psychotherapy sessions generally last?

Do not be fooled by the term "psychiatric hour." Most people would assume it means sixty minutes, but in fact most psychotherapy sessions run anywhere from forty-five to fifty minutes. Of course, if your therapist deems it useful to extend some sessions, then she will do so at her own discretion. For example, for a patient with severe depression and mania, the therapist might recommend briefer sessions several times a week if possible. For bipolar patients, the frequency of sessions is quite variable. Depending on the recommended course of treatment, you will see your therapist anywhere from once a day to once a month. Most psychiatrists and therapists agree that because bipolar disorder runs an unpredictable course, it is a good idea to stay in frequent touch as maintenance and coping issues arise.

How much will psychotherapy cost me?

The cost of psychotherapy is quite variable and is dependent on many factors. Some patients see their therapists in community mental health centers and outpatient clinics. Usually clinicians in these facilities charge clients on a sliding scale, depending on their income. Other patients see therapists who are in training at institutes and also pay on a sliding scale. Psychiatrists can charge anywhere from under a hundred dollars a session to well into the hundreds. Generally, psychiatrists, who are medical doctors, charge more than psychologists and social workers because they have trained longer and their credentials are more impressive. However, this is not always the case. Many psychologists and social workers also charge substantial fees for their services.

As insurance companies offer less and less coverage for mental health expenses, many clinicians have had to reduce their fees or lose patients. If you are interested in working with someone who you feel will make a big difference in your treatment but is too expensive, ask if there is any room for flexibility. There are no federal or state regulations regarding fees, and quite often clinicians are eager to create a situation that will meet everyone's needs. Keep in mind, however, that most clinicians will charge you for a missed session unless you call in advance and have a valid excuse.

Is therapy something I will look forward to, or will I dread my sessions?

This depends on many factors, including how you are feeling that day, how you have felt about therapy all along, what your relationship with your therapist is like, whether you think therapy is helping your condition, and whether you are depressed, hypomanic, or manic. Some days, your therapist's office will seem like the only place where you can breathe freely. On others you may resent the entire notion of the psychotherapeutic process, your therapist, and your illness. You are safe in assuming that your feelings will change over time and even from session to session. This is part of the normal process and is in keeping with the course of your condition and treatment. If you are unhappy going to therapy for an extended period of time, or even if you always look forward to it, it might be time to probe further into why. As hard as it may be, you may discover that you are uncomfortable with your current therapist. Though it is often difficult starting over with a new therapist, do not be afraid to search for a new practitioner if you feel you are no longer getting what you need from your current one. Before changing, however, obtain a second opinion from another doctor.

How do I know my therapist will keep everything I say confidential?

If your therapist has a thriving practice and has been treating patients for any length of time, it is doubtful that he or she does not respect patients' privacy. Psychiatrists, psychologists, and social workers, as well as anyone else working in medicine, go through extensive training to earn their degrees. Throughout their programs, supervisors and professors ingrain in them the importance of maintaining a client's confidentiality. Any therapist who betrays the confidence of his or her patients will soon find they have no referrals and will quickly be out of business.

The only time a clinician is obligated by law to break

a patient's confidentiality is when he deems the patient to be either suicidal or homicidal. Legally, morally, and ethically, the therapist must intervene by contacting the patient's family, a hospital, a rescue squad, or the police. If it seems feasible, the therapist should always give the patient the choice of voluntarily going to the hospital. If the patient refuses, the therapist is then forced to petition a court for an involuntary commitment to a care facility. Judging whether someone needs to be committed to a hospital against his will is an extremely difficult and almost always unpleasant task for a clinician. In the meantime, involving a family member or close friend to keep tabs on a potentially dangerous patient is a useful way to forestall any disasters.

How will I feel after my therapy sessions?

That depends on a number of factors, including:

- what you talked about during that particular session
- how you feel about your therapist
- how you are responding to the form of therapy your therapist is using
- your acceptance or denial of the illness
- how you feel that particular day about your work, family, etc.
- if you are having a hypomanic, manic, or depressive episode
- how well you are responding to your medication

You will probably feel a range of emotions, depending on the work you do during your session. It is not unusual to feel depressed, drained, and sad after discussing and working through some particularly difficult issues. On the other hand, you may have had a significant breakthrough about a problem that has been bothering you for some time, and, when you leave the session, you may feel like you have really made progress and are more in control of your life and the illness.

Psychotherapy is a process, and it generally takes time to feel the effects of all your hard work. Trusting that you will feel better over time, even if a specific session leaves you feeling down, is useful to keep in mind regarding psychotherapy. This is especially true for patients who have a chronic illness, like bipolar disorder, that continually changes and presents new challenges.

No matter how exhausting and depleting a session seems, you should still leave with the feeling that it had psychological value for you. Ultimately, the relationship with your therapist should remain one that is both positive and constructive.

How will psychotherapy help with my overall recovery?

Everyone responds to psychotherapy differently, depending on the specifics of his or her condition, the therapist, and the form of psychotherapy being used. Bipolar disorder, as we will discuss further in the following chapter, is something that clinicians need to treat primarily with medication. However, psychotherapy not only serves to help you understand the illness more comprehensively, but it may well enable you to live a happier and more fulfilling life. When it helps to reduce stress and combat the emotional upheavals that bipolar disorder often presents, psychotherapy is an excellent tool for maintaining control over your life.

Chapter 6

MEDICATION AND TREATING BIPOLAR DISORDER

Why do bipolar patients have to take medication?

Bipolar disorder results from the malfunctioning of the neurons (nerve cells) and the neurotransmitters (or "chemical messengers") involved in the mood centers of the brain. The disease manifests itself as a series of emotional and psychological disturbances and symptoms, but it derives mainly from physiological abnormalities. Understanding how to treat bipolar disorder with medication is a complicated task and a challenging area of study and research. Researchers and clinicians are continually discovering new agents for treating bipolar disorder, while at the same time fine-tuning medication regimens for optimal results and the fewest side effects.

Clinicians who prescribe and monitor bipolar medications have to be informed and skilled practitioners. The medications are complicated, and each individual responds to them differently. Generally, though, the drugs are both safe and effective when administered correctly. Not surprisingly, it is the patients who do not comply with prescribed regimens of medication who tend to have the poorest results.

When did doctors start treating mania with medication?

As always with bipolar disorder, clinicians must combat the illness in different ways, depending on whether the patient is manic or depressed. But they must always bear in mind that the manic patient may become depressed and, perhaps more important, that the depressed patient may become manic. The paradox in treating a bipolar patient with medication is that the clinician is really treating two diseases at once, but this has only come to light in the past few decades.

Lithium, the "gold standard" of antimanic medications for the past forty years or so, was the first modern medication clinicians gave to bipolar patients. After World War II, Australian physician John Cade discovered lithium's therapeutic value while experimenting with guinea pigs. His observations and discoveries were not fully recognized in Europe until the mid-1950s, when Mogens Schou of Denmark confirmed Cade's earlier work. A few American psychiatrists used lithium during the fifties, but it was not widely prescribed here until the late 1960s.

A small group of clinicians began using anticonvulsant drugs to treat mania in the early 1970s. Today, doctors commonly use medications such as Tegretol and Depakote (both FDA approved), which continue to show excellent therapeutic promise for manic patients. In fact, clinicians often prescribe Depakote as a "first-line" (first-choice) medication instead of lithium. Additionally, patients tend to suffer fewer side effects with anticonvulsants than they do with lithium.

What progress has been made by the medical community and the pharmaceutical industry in treating bipolar depression?

Debate continues to rage over the importance of studying the differences between unipolar and bipolar depressions. Overall, the treatment of severe depression in recent decades has been nothing short of revolutionary. In addition to effective medication treatments, the use of electroconvulsive therapy (ECT), which we will discuss further in chapter 7, has been honed and refined. The hopelessness, despondency, and sadness that is at

the very core of depression can now be alleviated more
effectively and more quickly than at any other time in
the history of mental illness treatment. However, while
the general treatment for unipolar depression has pro-
gressed at a rapid pace, the study and development of
medications specifically for bipolar depression has,
sadly, been lagging behind.

The most vexing aspect of treating bipolar depression is the possibility of inducing mania or rapid cycling. Many bipolar patients are excluded from new
antidepressant medication trials because of their tendency to become manic.

Currently, researchers are testing the efficacy of antimanic agents as antidepressants as well. John Cade
and researchers after him found that lithium had very
little antidepressant effect, and in some cases worsened
the patient's depression. Combining certain antidepressants with antimanic agents for a limited amount of
time is an option that many clinicians are now seriously
investigating.

How will my doctor determine if I need medication?

Diagnosing your illness correctly is the first step your
doctor must make toward medicating you properly. As
we have discussed in previous chapters, determining
whether you have bipolar disorder is not always simple,
because there are many extenuating circumstances that
can lead to an improper diagnosis. Your doctor will
begin by taking a comprehensive psychiatric and medical history that includes:

1. History of depressive or manic episodes: their
   length, when they first occurred, and the severity of
   the symptoms
2. Your age at the time of the first episode
3. Any other medical conditions you may have or
   have had
4. Any prior treatments for psychiatric or physical

conditions, where you were treated, and who treated you

5. Any prior hospitalizations
6. Any prior suicide attempts or violent behavior
7. Family history of relatives with bipolar disorder, unipolar depression, or alcoholism

If you are unable to provide your doctor with all the information she needs, then she should ask a family member or one of your close friends for help.

Once your doctor has determined that you do in fact have bipolar disorder, she will begin another series of tests to determine your present psychological and physical condition.

The term "psychiatric exam" sounds a little scary. What will my doctor ask me?

A psychiatric exam can consist of little more than a psychiatrist or a psychologist making observations and asking you questions. But when a doctor is trying to determine whether or not you should be medicated for an illness like bipolar disorder, the exam might be a little more complicated.

The exam generally follows these guidelines:

• The doctor will ask you a number of questions and observe your general appearance and behavior in an attempt to determine your mood.

• The doctor will assess your general orientation—for example, asking you "Do you know where you are? and "What time of the year is it?"

• He will also want to know the content (the "what") and the process (the "how") of your thoughts. That is to say, can you communicate your thoughts clearly, are they sequential and rational or completely disorganized, and are you having difficulty expressing yourself? The doctor will want to know if you have had any delusions (false beliefs), and he will observe if your speech is pressured (too rapid and fast).

- Determining whether your symptoms are due to another medical problem requires the doctor to test your cognitive and intellectual functioning. He can do this partially during the psychiatric exam by testing, for example, your memory or ability to perform simple calculations. The doctor is also looking for a number of medical conditions, such as Alzheimer's disease and acute drug intoxication.
- Finally, the doctor will assess if your judgment and insight are sound.

You are more likely to answer these questions if you are depressed or have been stabilized after either a manic or depressive episode. If you are currently manic, you may be unable to answer in a rational manner and the doctor or medical team will assess the need for medication based on their observations. For example, if you have been brought into a hospital by a medical emergency team because you have been threatening to kill your mother and then yourself with a knife, a psychiatrist will probably first administer an antipsychotic drug like Haldol to calm you down. Once you are less aggressive, then the psychiatrist can more easily determine why you became psychotic.

How important is it for my doctors to know about prior bipolar episodes when trying to medicate me?

It is crucial that any doctor trying to treat you get, if possible, a detailed history of all prior episodes you have had, if they occurred after a stressful life event, and how severe they were. Additionally, he will ask if you had a positive reaction, an adverse one, or if the medication had no effect on your condition. If you have had a negative response to an antidepressant, for example, it may have led to poor compliance on your part. Learning how you once responded to medications, psychotherapy, and changes in your life can be extremely helpful to doctors in creating a successful medication plan for the future.

If you or your family has kept any written or recorded documentation regarding past episodes, make copies for your current doctor. You can have medical records sent to your new physician by calling any hospital or doctor's office where you were once treated. If this is too great a task for you, ask a family member or friend to make the calls. If you do have a past history of bipolar episodes, your doctor will greatly appreciate any records that come into his possession.

Will my doctor want to know if anyone in my family has taken medication for a mental illness?

Yes. In addition to taking a thorough history of any mental illness in your immediate or extended family, your doctor will also want to know about family response to medication. Studies show that if, for example, your mother has bipolar disorder and responds well to a particular antimanic medication, there is a good chance that you will too. By learning how your family members responded, doctors can also surmise how you might respond to certain combinations of drugs and what side effects you might suffer.

Will I have to take physical tests before my doctor prescribes medication?

First you will undergo a battery of physical tests to:

1. Rule out the possibility that your mania is due to any other medical conditions or chemical substances (e.g., cocaine or amphetamine abuse, brain infection, or depression because of a thyroid problem or anemia)

2. Make sure that it is medically safe for you to take the prescribed medication (e.g., that your liver can break down the drug and your kidneys can eliminate it)

The initial physical exam, which is reasonably standard, will begin with the basics: height, weight, reflexes, listening to your chest, eyes, ears, nose, throat, and blood pressure. The doctor uses the results from the following tests to rule out the possibility of a "mimicking" disorder (e.g., thyroid disease, anemia, etc.) and to ensure the safety of using certain medications.

The tests include:

1. Blood work (e.g., to check red and white blood cell counts)
2. "Chem screen" (which includes testing kidney and liver function, and blood salts)
3. Urinalysis to check for normal kidney function
4. Thyroid profile
5. Electrocardiogram (EKG) to test condition of the heart
6. The occasional central nervous system or radiological exam (e.g., CAT scan or MRI)

Some tests may cause you a bit of initial discomfort, but ultimately it is better for your doctor to understand as much about your physical condition as she can before prescribing any medications.

If I feel unsure about the medication plan my doctor presents, can I seek a second opinion?

Absolutely. If you or a family member ever feels unsure about something, ask your doctor about her choices. If her answer does not satisfy you, seek another opinion. However, it may not be necessary to change doctors. You may feel more comfortable obtaining a second opinion, but maintaining continuity with one doctor is very important. Obviously, if you do not trust or like your doctor, finding another one is necessary, but do not stop seeing the first doctor until you have found another. One option is to have the second doctor communicate your concerns and offer feedback to your current doctor. Ideally, you can stay with the first and benefit from the input of the second.

A sign that it may be time to consult with someone else is this: You find your current medication regimen is not working for you and your doctor is reluctant to change your prescriptions. Everyone responds differently to the numerous medications available today, and your doctor might be missing something that another one will be able to figure out.

It is helpful to keep in mind that medicating a bipolar patient is not an easy or straightforward task. There are many variables involved, and it may take time to hit upon the combination of factors (medication, psychotherapy, lifestyle modifications) that is just right for you. You should try to avoid making drastic changes and should always seek the support of your family and friends before making any decisions.

What are the phases of treatment for bipolar disorder?

Once again, the duality of bipolar disorder becomes apparent in the treatment of the two major phases of the illness. The first phase involves dealing with the acute or current aspects of the illness. This involves stabilizing a manic patient who has just been admitted to the hospital or helping a depressed patient feel like it is worth getting up and going to work every day. Both of these examples are treatable with medication, but clinicians have to take great care to ensure the proper dosage, monitoring, and compliance. Bipolar patients are most vulnerable in the throes of an episode, and the overall goal is to get them to feel and function normally as quickly as possible.

During the second phase, patients and their doctors work toward preventing future episodes of the illness. Maintaining a regimen of medication and learning to identify early warning symptoms are important elements in living with bipolar disorder. When learning how to tolerate the effects of certain maintenance drugs, such as lithium, patients have to work with their doctors and medical team. For most patients, bipolar disorder is a chronic illness that often requires the ongoing use of medications. Taking these maintenance medications is not always easy, and there are several issues that both patients and doctors have to consider before establishing a plan.

What are some of the issues my doctor and I should discuss before I begin taking medication?

There are dozens of factors that your doctor or medical team will consider, ask about, and advise you on before medication treatment begins. As with most medications, there are several basic issues that warrant discussion. These include:

- How the medication will react with alcohol
- How the medication will react with prescription and over-the-counter drugs
- If the medication is safe for pregnant or nursing women
- If you will be able to drive or operate machinery while taking the medication
- If you have any allergies
- Your age (medications work differently on children and the elderly)
- If you will need to be monitored daily, weekly, monthly, or yearly
- How the medications for bipolar disorder will react with other drugs you may be taking for other conditions
- If you are taking herbs or other alternative substances, how the medications will interact with these somewhat unknown quantities
- If you will need to have blood work performed regularly. If so, at what intervals?
- How long it will take for the medication to take effect initially

- If you stop taking your medication, how long it will take to be effective once you resume treatment
- If you are taking more than one medication, what the side effects are separately and together
- Where you can find information regarding studies of new medications
- What the out-of-pocket cost will be to you and your family for the medications

By making a list of all the questions you and your family want answers to, you can significantly affect both the initial and long-term course of your illness. You can never have too much information regarding your treatment, and every day there is more new and encouraging material to add to your storehouse of knowledge.

Why is it important for me to work closely with my doctor when taking medication?

Medication treatments for bipolar disorder are becoming increasingly varied and more successful. However, it is still an ever-changing and ongoing process. The most effective way to treat the illness is for you and your family to develop a close relationship and open dialogue with your doctor. He must carefully follow your progress by assessing both the benefits of medications as well as their side effects. Many medications require occasional to frequent blood tests that your doctor will use to determine what modifications he needs to make in your treatment. Your doctor, or the doctor who covers for him when he is not working or on "call," should be available to you and your family twenty-four hours a day. Do not hesitate to call with questions and concerns, especially if it is an emergency.

Many patients are discouraged that some medications do not work immediately and can take weeks to become effective. In addition, both mania and depression can distort your sense of time and make you feel like the medication will never work. Before you consider making any changes in your treatment or decide to stop taking medications, speak to your doctor. He will probably tell you that if you are a "patient" patient and trust him, you will feel better shortly.

What is a mood stabilizer?

Mood stabilizers are the cornerstones in the treatment of bipolar disorder. These medications, which include lithium, Depakote, and Tegretol, effectively treat mania and block the recurrence of both mania and depression. In addition, some have mild to modest antidepressant properties. The use of mood stabilizers as antidepressants is extremely beneficial to those patients prone to swinging from depression to mania.

The three principal mood stabilizers currently used in the treatment of mania are:

1. *Lithium carbonate (Eskalith, Lithobid, Carbolith, Lithane, Duralith, and others):* This pioneering medication in the treatment of mania is the one against which all others are compared. It may be best used now, experts believe, in patients with a later age onset (generally twenty-five years or older). Lithium may also benefit bipolar patients with impaired psychosocial functioning. While it is effective in 60 to 80 percent of all hypomanic and manic episodes, experts are not sure of its mechanism. Some researchers theorize that lithium may stabilize membranes around neurons and decrease the excitability of nerves around mood centers. Lithium may take weeks to become effective in patients, so clinicians generally do not use it for the immediate treatment of mixed and rapid cycling states.

2. *Valproate (Depakote, Depakene):* Formerly used exclusively for the treatment of epilepsy, this anticonvulsant is a good alternative for patients who do not respond to lithium. Currently, experts recommend a combined program of lithium and valproate for treating acute manic episodes. Both valproate and carbamazepine, another anticonvulsant used as a mood stabilizer,

may stimulate the activity of a "quieting" neuro-transmitter called gaba-aminobutyric acid (GABA). Valproate and carbamazepine may also work as an "anti-kindling" agent by keeping neurons from overfir-ing. Patients appear to be at a higher risk for a break-through depression (meaning that symptoms can develop even when you are taking medication) with val-proate than with lithium. Valproate may also be more effective with younger patients suffering the onset of the disorder, and those who experience mixed and rapid cycling states. This drug is the only other mood stabi-lizer on the market besides lithium that has been ap-proved by the FDA for use in treating bipolar disorder. However, that does not mean that doctors cannot pre-scribe other medications at their discretion. One of the more serious side effects of valproate that doctors must watch for is liver inflammation.

3. *Carbamazepine (Tegretol):* Carbamazepine is also used for epilepsy and has been found to be an effective mood stabilizer. For patients who do not respond well to lithium alone, experts recommend that doctors try combinations of carbamazepine, valproate, and lithium. Of course, this should be done only after the patient has been thoroughly tested for possible adverse reactions. Studies have shown that taken in combination these drugs more quickly reduce the amount of time a person stays in the hospital after an acute episode as compared with those patients given lithium alone. Doctors should always watch for a potential lowering of blood counts in patients. FDA approval for this drug is pending.

Are there more mood stabilizers available for treatment?

Yes. Lithium, valproate (from here on referred to as Depakote), and carbamazepine (from here on referred to as Tegretol) are currently the three most effective mood stabilizers, but there are several other medica-tions available to clinicians.

   Listed below are other agents that may be of use in the treatment of bipolar disorder:

   1. *Clonazepam (Klonopin):* A physician may administer this anticonvulsant medication if a manic patient is experiencing symptoms, such as severe agitation, in conjunction with one of the mood stabilizers previously discussed. Clonazepam, a Valium-type drug, is very useful for agitated patients because it has a rapid calming effect. It is generally not used once the mood-stabilizing effects of lithium, Depakote, or Tegretol take hold. One of the positive aspects of this medication is that it requires no blood monitoring and can be safely used in combination with many other substances. Beyond just being a sedative, clonazepam may also have specific antimanic properties (e.g., it may prevent further manic episodes) for some patients. In addition to clonazepam, another benzodiazepine (antianxiety medication) that clinicians administer to manic patients is lorazepam (Ativan).

   2. *Gabapentin (Neurontin):* Gabapentin is known to be helpful in controlling epileptic seizures and now shows great promise as a mood stabilizer as well. Currently, it is more commonly used as an adjunct to other mood stabilizers. Gabapentin has very positive antianxiety properties, and clinicians are beginning to use it to calm patients.

   3. *Lamotrigine (Lamictal):* Lamotrigine, also an anticonvulsant, appears to work very well as a mood stabilizer, but it is mostly used now as an adjunct to other medications. Lamotrigine seems to have antidepressant properties, but it can cause a potentially life-threatening rash. Patients who take this anticonvulsant need to be monitored very closely by a medical professional.

What are calcium channel blockers and how do they affect manic patients?

Clinicians use calcium channel blockers mainly to treat hypertension. The medications affect the movement of calcium into the cells of the heart and blood vessels. By relaxing the blood vessels, they increase the supply of blood and oxygen to the heart and reduce its workload. By alleviating pressure on the heart and arteries, calcium channel blockers can limit damage done to blood vessels of the brain, heart, and kidneys. If your blood pressure is under control, you are less likely to suffer strokes, heart failure, and kidney failure.

Several studies have found that when a person is manic, their calcium levels are altered. Experts now suggest that calcium channel blockers, such as nimodipine (Nimotop) and verapamil (Calan), may have depressant, tranquilizing, and antimanic effects. One study reported that verapamil was as effective on manic patients as neuroleptics, or a neuroleptic and lithium combination, with much fewer side effects. Many clinicians are moving ahead of researchers and prescribing calcium channel blockers for mania, thus creating a need to study the medications further. As of this writing, it does appear that Neurontin and Lamictal will be more effective as antimanic agents than Nimotop and Calan.

Researchers have also discovered that one of the biological mechanisms involved with rapid cycling is an increased amount of calcium movement into brain cells. Nimotop, a calcium channel blocker, is proving to be very beneficial for patients who experience rapid cycling.

If you are pregnant or breast-feeding, it is probably not advisable to take calcium channel blockers, as there is not enough data on their effects to fetuses and babies. Calcium channel blockers can interact with other medications—beta-blockers or Tegretol, for example—in adverse ways, so it is very important that your doctor know all of the medications you are currently taking. Side effects that can result from taking calcium channel blockers include drowsiness, weight gain, constipation, and diarrhea.

Why do medications often have more than one name?

Medications generally have one generic name, but many have several brand names. The brand name is given to the drug by whichever company manufactures and distributes it. For example, amitriptyline is the generic name for a tricyclic antidepressant medication. Elavil and Endep are different brand names for the same drug. As a rule, generic names begin with a lowercase letter, while brand names begin with a capital letter. For the most part in this book, we refer to medications by their brand names, since more people are familiar with these names than their generic counterparts. However, since there are a great number of brand names for lithium and most people know it only by the generic name, we will refer to all lithium drugs simply as "lithium."

What is the difference between benzodiazepine and neuroleptic medications?

Benzodiazepines, like Klonopin and Ativan, are antianxiety drugs generally used to sedate agitated patients. They are helpful for bipolar patients having manic episodes who need to be stabilized but are uncooperative and anxious. Neuroleptics, which professionals divide into atypical and typical groupings, are antipsychotic medications, like haloperidol (Haldol), chlorpromazine (Thorazine), and clozapine (Clozaril). The properties of these medications make them very helpful for patients with psychotic symptoms such as delusions. Neuroleptics, especially typical ones, may cause a significant side effect called *tardive dyskinesia*. The effect is characterized by abnormal body movements, usually of the arms, mouth, and tongue. Most experts feel that clinicians should use benzodiazepines before administering neuroleptics. Once the acute manic symptoms pass, clinicians usually discontinue using both benzodiazepines and neuroleptics.

How do "typical" and "atypical" neuroleptics differ?

Neuroleptics as a class of medications are used by clinicians to treat psychotic disorders, such as schizophrenia. They have the ability to both initially sedate and then calm a patient suffering an acute manic episode. However, it now appears that atypical neuroleptics may be more effective for treating some bipolar patients. Additionally, the atypicals seem to produce fewer side effects, more selectively block some dopamine receptors, and have effects on serotonin levels; also, they may reduce persistent psychotic symptoms. Both types need to be studied further to truly understand their potential effects on bipolar patients.

The atypical neuroleptics include:

- clozapine (Clozaril)
- olanzapine (Zyprexa)
- quetiapine (Seroquel)
- risperidone (Risperdal)

The typical neuroleptics include:

- chlorpromazine (Thorazine)
- fluphenazine (Prolixin)
- haloperidol (Haldol)
- loxapine (Loxitane)
- mesoridazine (Serentil)
- molindine (Moban)
- perphenazine (Trilafon)
- thioridazine (Mellaril)
- thiothixene (Navane)
- trifluoperazine (Stelazine)

Significantly, there is no need for blood level monitoring with neuroleptics or, for that matter, with Neurontin and Lamictal. However, with lithium, Depakote, and Tegretol, patients must initially have blood levels checked every week. Once the patient is stabilized, clinicians check levels every month and eventually several times a year.

Is there any instance where neuroleptics and anticonvulsants work better than lithium?

Many experts now believe that for the first week or two of an acute manic episode, both neuroleptics and anticonvulsants work more quickly for the bipolar patient than lithium because of their sedative effect. After the first two weeks, lithium and, for example, Depakote and Tegretol are more effective than neuroleptics. The two anticonvulsants can take anywhere from four days to two weeks to take effect. Obviously, when a patient does not respond to lithium, Depakote, or Tegretol treatments, or cannot tolerate their effects, neuroleptics and the other medications mentioned above (e.g., Klonopin and Ativan) are the best possible alternatives.

Do doctors ever use hormones to treat mania?

Some clinicians have used high doses of thyroid hormone, generally T4 (Synthroid) in conjunction with other medications. During the maintenance phase of bipolar disorder, T4 is sometimes used by clinicians to maintain normal moods. More commonly used to correct low thyroid functioning, these drugs have met with mixed results.

What are the side effects of lithium?

One of the greatest drawbacks to lithium treatment is that only slightly elevated blood levels of the medication can cause significant side effects and toxicity. Maintaining just the right amount of lithium in the blood is essential. During acute attacks, levels must be checked frequently, and about every three months during the maintenance phase. Patients on lithium should drink two to three quarts of water a day, use normal amounts of salt, and avoid dehydration at all costs. Clinicians use the measurement mEq/L to specify levels of lithium in the blood. Safe levels are usually 0.5 to 1.2 mEq/L during the initial treatment and 0.5 to 1 mEq/L for maintenance therapy.

Side effects include:

1. Metallic taste in the mouth
2. Sedation
3. Thirst
4. Hand tremors
5. Nausea

Certain people can tolerate higher blood levels than others without ill effects. However, for most people, if levels of lithium are even slightly elevated in the blood, toxic reactions can occur. Some of the side effects of high levels of lithium include confusion, severe trembling, nausea, an increase in urine output, and loss of coordination. For higher levels of toxicity, more severe reactions involve convulsions, uncontrolled movements of arms and legs, blurred vision, nausea and vomiting, stupor, and sometimes coma. Blood levels over 2.5 mEq/L are very dangerous and can be fatal.

Fortunately, physicians check blood levels frequently and can adjust dosages for their patients as needed. Patients taking lithium or their family members should always alert a medical professional at the first sign of any unusual symptoms.

Are there any medical conditions or medications that can affect levels of lithium in the blood?

Actually, there are several that patients should be aware of, including high fever, diabetes, dieting, salt-restrictive diets, and diarrhea. Lithium is eliminated from the body through the kidneys, so any drugs that affect kidney functioning may alter levels in the blood. Some medications that may affect the amount of lithium in the blood are:

- nonsteroidal anti-inflammatory drugs (NSAIDs) (e.g., aspirin)
- thiazide diuretics (for high blood pressure or fluid retention)
- ACE inhibitors
- hypertension and congestive heart failure drugs (calcium channel blockers)
- antipsychotics
- anticonvulsants

Overall, the risk associated with these medications is low, but physicians still need to be cautious.

Researchers are conducting studies on how seasonal change may affect lithium levels. For example, one study found that levels are higher in men in the summer, which means lower doses may be necessary for men during these months. Another study involving gastric lavage, a stomach-rinsing procedure, may be useful for treating overdoses of lithium. It should be noted, however, that studies and procedures like these are still in the preliminary stages.

What are some of the long-term effects of lithium usage?

Patients often become exhausted from dealing with the side effects and monitoring of lithium. Additionally, many patients crave the energy and optimism that accompanied their mania. One study illustrated the reality of widespread noncompliance by showing that patients took their medication an astoundingly low 34 percent of the time. Another found that about a third of bipolar patients eventually stopped taking the drug altogether.

Some of the uncomfortable side effects that patients report are:

- weight gain
- hair loss
- unpleasant taste in mouth

- skin eruptions resembling acne
- worsening of psoriasis (dry skin condition)
- loss of sex drive
- thyroid problems
- impaired kidney functioning (may be dangerous)
- memory loss
- dulled emotions
- slow mental functioning
- lack of motor coordination
- reduced sensitivity to light
- slightly affected color recognition
- problems with night driving

Some experts recommend that patients being treated with lithium wear sunglasses and avoid intense exposure to bright light for extended periods of time.

Taking lithium entails a constant weighing of pros and cons. Remember, experts have been treating bipolar patients with lithium for more than forty years. For most patients, the drug is effective and safe when administered by an informed and skilled practitioner. Most physicians feel that patients can continue to take lithium over the course of a lifetime.

What are the side effects of Depakote?

Clinicians formerly used Depakote as an alternative for bipolar patients who either did not respond to or could not tolerate lithium. For reasons still unknown, somewhere between 20 and 40 percent of bipolar patients do not respond to lithium treatment. Currently, experts are encouraging the use of combinations of the anticonvulsants with lithium, with each other, or on their own.

In clinical studies, Depakote appears to have relatively minor side effects, which tend to occur early in treatment and then subside. Some patients have gastrointestinal (GI) problems, including nausea, vomiting, and heartburn. Patients also report:

- headaches
- vision problems
- ringing in the ears
- hair loss
- weight gain
- agitation
- odd motor movements
- menstrual irregularities
- increase in risk of polycystic ovaries

Notably, Depakote is recommended for women taking oral contraceptives, but it greatly increases the risk of birth defects if taken during pregnancy. Rare but serious side effects relating to Depakote are liver damage, convulsions, and, in some instances, coma.

What are the side effects of Tegretol?

Like Depakote, Tegretol is now found to be most beneficial for refractory (generally nonresponsive to medication) bipolar patients when taken in combination with lithium. Tegretol's side effects, not surprisingly, are quite similar to those of Depakote. Weight gain, hair loss, and tremors appear to be more pronounced with Depakote than Tegretol, but Tegretol can produce far more dangerous skin reactions. About 6 percent of patients taking Tegretol have such severe skin reactions to the drug that they have to discontinue using it.

Roughly 10 percent of patients who take Tegretol experience a decrease in white blood cells. This is usually not very serious unless the individual has an infection or a weakened immune system. There are some other blood conditions that can occur, and patients should always tell their doctor if they develop a sore throat, fever, easy bruising, or unusual bleeding. Owing to the risk of birth defects, pregnant women should not take Tegretol. In elderly patients, water retention can be a problem.

How do doctors treat pregnant women with bipolar disorder?

Past studies have shown that women who take lithium during the first three months of pregnancy have an increased risk of delivering babies with heart and other birth defects. More recently, though, research in this area indicates that taking lithium may be safer than was formerly believed. It is still advisable to weigh the risks of prescribing lithium during pregnancy against new data. Some physicians now cautiously administer lithium near the time of delivery, believing that both mother and child are out of danger. Women who take lithium after their child is born should not breast-feed, as lithium concentrates in breast milk.

Women with bipolar disorder are at a great risk for developing mania directly after giving birth (one study found that 20 percent of women were hospitalized within ninety days after delivery). If a woman takes mood stabilizers at the time of delivery, her risk substantially decreases, but practitioners must take great care with monitoring and follow through in these cases.

As mentioned earlier, anticonvulsants increase the chance for physical malformations, developmental delays, and spina bifida in infants and should *never* be taken during pregnancy.

If possible, mild manic episodes during pregnancy should be treated without the use of drugs. If absolutely necessary, doctors can use typical antipsychotic medications, like Thorazine, with severely disturbed patients. The most effective treatment for a woman with bipolar disorder having an acute manic episode during pregnancy appears to be electroconvulsive therapy (ECT). We will look at this form of treatment in chapter 7.

How does the medication treatment of children and adolescents differ from that of adults?

Experts now realize that mania and mania-like states occur more frequently in adolescents and even prepubescent children than previously believed (or thought by clinicians). Clinicians aim to treat these episodes as quickly as possible so as to prevent their severity and the number of subsequent episodes. In addition, the emotional and social scars that these episodes leave on children and adolescents can take a great toll. The idea is that the sooner practitioners treat the illness, the better the patient's long-term prospects.

With lithium, the same course of treatment that experts prescribe for adults generally is effective for younger people. Some studies report that children may respond even better to lithium treatment than adults. However, some early onsets of the illness indicate more mixed and rapid cycling states, which tend to require anticonvulsant treatment as well as lithium. Blood levels and side effects seem nearly the same for children as adults, taking into account adjustments for weight and overall size. Unfortunately, getting children to comply with medication can be very difficult. Concerns about peer pressure, weight gain, acne, and other side effects of the drug treatment often create resistance.

In the first week of treatment, children under age six who are given lithium tend to have severe side effects, generally related to the central nervous system. Only physicians who are very experienced with the effects of lithium on children this young should ever prescribe the medication for them.

Adolescents go through a number of hormonal changes and tend to experiment with chemical substances that can affect reactions to medication. How both of these factors affect their overall response to bipolar medications is an area that needs further study and evaluation.

How are the elderly treated for mania?

Mania in the elderly is often difficult to diagnose because of concurrent symptoms stemming from such disorders as organic brain syndrome. Clinicians have to carefully consider whether an elderly person's mania is caused by some medical condition or medication other than bipolar disorder. This is especially true if the person has never had a manic episode before. Once the clinician finds that the mania is not related to any other condition, she should treat the patient with antimanic medications. The next challenge is to determine whether the medication will interact adversely with other existing medical problems and drugs.

While the data is not complete, there is some evidence that suggests that medication-related side effects are more severe in the elderly. This could relate to, for example, generally compromised renal functioning and overall health. Older patients may be more sensitive to neurotoxic effects of antimanic drugs and vulnerable to tardive dyskinesia (especially patients taking neuroleptics).

Are there any formulas that doctors use to determine dosage?

Yes. There are several mathematical formulas, based on body weight and other factors that doctors use to determine dosages. Once the doctor has calculated the proper amount of medication for a patient, he must consider how long the drug takes to become effective. Lithium takes about four to ten days to take effect; Depakote works much faster—it often has an onset within seventy-two hours of being administered and is very useful for mixed and rapid cycling states. Sometimes clinicians give patients a "loading dose" of medication, meaning that they do not gradually increase amounts but give the entire dose from the initiation of treatment for a quicker response.

If I'm having an acute manic episode, how will my doctor determine what dose of a medication to give me?

Determining how much of a medication a patient needs is an ongoing challenge for the practitioner. Patients and their physicians must keep in constant communication about the positive effects and side effects of medications. Doctors can also gain helpful information from both frequent and periodic blood tests.

Dosage considerations for antimanic agents are as follows:

1. *Lithium:* There is an extremely narrow gap between levels of lithium that are therapeutic and those that are toxic. However, clinicians can easily determine blood levels and have studied required doses quite extensively. For acute mania, experts recommend the highest dose possible without harmful side effects until the patient is stabilized. Maintenance dosage levels are substantially lower. The dose-to-blood-level ratio is determined by an individual patient's:

- sex
- age
- weight (especially muscle mass)
- salt intake
- perspiration levels
- intrinsic renal clearance for lithium
- other medications

A somewhat higher dose-to-blood-level ratio is associated with young, heavy male patients who have a high salt intake. In general, greater amounts of lithium are needed to achieve optimal blood levels in manic patients than in those who are euthymic or depressed. As a patient's mania subsides, doctors decrease lithium dosages to avoid a possible toxic reaction. Clinicians monitor blood levels more closely during these times when a patient's clinical profile is in flux. This is especially true when going from mania to euthymia or depression.

2. *Neuroleptics:* Formerly, clinicians used very high doses of neuroleptics for acute mania, but they have found that in most cases more modest amounts are equally effective. Doctors consider clinical state, age, gender, and weight when determining required dosages

of medications. If the patient is young, male, heavy, and extremely disturbed, doses will probably be higher than those prescribed for other patients. As an example of neuroleptic dosages, practitioners usually start patients on 1 to 5 mg of Haldol intramuscularly or 2 to 10 mg orally every 4 to 6 hours. The recommended dose of Thorazine, on the other hand, is 25 to 100 mg intramuscularly every 4 hours, which is then gradually replaced by oral doses. Clinicians should constantly reevaluate the need for neuroleptics during an acute manic phase and taper them as symptoms begin to subside.

3. *Tegretol:* When given alone, the initial dose of Tegretol is usually 200 to 400 mg. The dose is then increased, based on blood levels, to somewhere between 800 to 1,000 mg during the first week. If combined with lithium or neuroleptics, the dosage and target blood level are generally somewhat lower. Side effects are more likely to occur if dosages of Tegretol are administered more rapidly, as when treating acute mania. They are less likely during the prophylactic phase, when the dosage builds up more slowly.

4. *Depakote:* During an acute manic phase, Depakote is often used as a first-line drug instead of lithium. The dosage generally starts at 500 to 1,500 mg/day in divided doses. There appear to be very few adverse effects, and side effects are either minimal or completely absent. However, when Depakote is combined with Tegretol, clinicians should monitor blood levels frequently, as the two medications interact with each other in metabolically complicated ways.

How do clinicians treat bipolar depression with medication?

There are a number of similarities between treating a bipolar patient for depression and treating her for mania, but there are many differences as well. Even if the patient does not appear to be spiraling out of control, as many patients do in mania, the welfare of the depressed patient is no less serious. Unaware that a patient is in fact bipolar, a clinician may induce a manic episode by prescribing antidepressants for depression. As we have stated several times in this book, clinicians must make a careful examination of a patient before administering medication. This includes finding out if there have been any past bipolar episodes and if there is a history of bipolar disorder in the family. Information regarding past hypomanic and manic episodes frequently has to come from family members, as the depressed patient is often unable to judge the severity of prior episodes. The timing, however, can be crucial, especially if the patient is suicidal.

What are some of the pertinent historical facts that clinicians will want to know before beginning medication?

The facts include:

- how old the patient was when he had his first depressive, hypomanic, or manic episode
- characteristics of each prior episode: severity, duration, nature of symptoms, and if there was any pattern of recurrence (e.g., seasonal onset)
- how the patient responded to any prior medications. This is very important, because sometimes the only indication of bipolar disorder is a brief hypomanic period following the use of antidepressants.
- how family members have responded to antidepressants, since relatives often respond to medications in similar ways

Are bipolar patients treated any differently from unipolar patients?

Generally, bipolar patients who are depressed are treated with the same medications as those given to patients with unipolar depression. The primary difference is that an attempt is made to keep the bipolar patient from swinging into a manic phase. Doctors do this by putting patients on a mood stabilizer before they administer any antidepressants. Sometimes all the patient needs is the mood stabilizer to alleviate the depressive symptoms. Additionally, a patient needs medication when his depression does not respond to external events, such as changing jobs or engaging in psychotherapy. Disturbances in mood, sleep, and appetite are also good indicators for drug treatment. Many experts feel that more research needs to be done on the biological and clinical differences between bipolar and unipolar depression. If researchers find appreciable differences, then clinicians may be able to address the specific needs of bipolar depression more efficiently and quickly.

Are there any specific approaches to treating bipolar depression?

Clinicians often use a model called a "drug decision tree" to outline treatment for bipolar depression. They can also apply the decision tree to patients having a mixed episode.

For bipolar depression, the drug decision tree begins with a mood stabilizer, such as lithium, Depakote, or Tegretol. Doctors also give these medications in combination if they appear to be more effective that way. Next, an antidepressant is necessary for relieving depressive symptoms. The antidepressants are for the most part equally effective, but certain drugs should never be combined with others. For example, an MAOI like Nardil or Parnate should rarely if ever be used with another antidepressant. Doctors must add the antidepressant slowly and carefully to avoid mania. If the patient does not respond to one antidepressant, another should be tried.

The decision tree continues with suggestions for additional or alternative medications, such as the anticonvulsants Lamictal and Neurontin or the thyroid medication thyroxine (Synthroid and others). The final portion of the tree encourages clinicians to use electroconvulsive therapy (ECT) when medications are not effective or patients are intolerant of them.

How long should a bipolar patient stay on antidepressants?

Generally, clinicians recommend that unipolar patients stay on antidepressants after a first episode anywhere from four to nine months once their overt symptoms have disappeared. For bipolar depression, a mood stabilizer is a doctor's first choice for medication. Patients who respond well to a mood stabilizer alone after a first episode should stay on their medication for about a year. Patients who have two or more episodes should probably continue on their medication for an indefinite period of time. Depending on how patients respond, they and the doctor should discuss the possibility of slowly and carefully tapering the medication.

Patients who need to take an antidepressant during a first episode of bipolar depression should stay on the drug for four to nine months. They should take the antidepressant only if the drug has been shown to have positive effects on their condition. With two or more episodes, the length of time for antidepressants is more open-ended. Currently, there is no hard data on when to taper antidepressants after multiple depressive episodes.

Which antidepressants do clinicians use for treating bipolar depression?

The antidepressants include:

1. *Monoamine oxidase inhibitors (MAOIs):*

   - phenelzine (Nardil)
   - tranylcypromine (Parnate)

2. *Tricyclic antidepressants:*

   - amitriptyline (Elavil, and others)

- clomipramine (Anafranil)
- desipramine (Norpramin, Pertofrane)
- doxepin (Adapine, Sienquan)
- imipramine (Tofranil)
- nortriptyline (Vivactil)
- trimipramine (Surmontil)

3. *Selective serotonin reuptake inhibitors (SSRIs):*

- citalopram (Celexa)
- fluoxetine (Prozac)
- fluvoxamine (Luvox)
- paroxetine (Paxil)
- sertraline (Zoloft)

4. *Tetracyclic antidepressants:*

- amoxapine (Asendin)
- maprotiline (Ludiomil)

5. *Novel or heterocyclic antidepressants:*

- bupropion (Wellbutrin)
- mirtazapine (Remeron)
- nefazodone (Serzone)
- trazodone (Desyrel)
- venlafaxine (Effexor)

For a more complete description of these medications and the use of antidepressants, see *If You Think You Have Depression,* also Dell's Guide for Mental Health series.

Are certain antidepressants more effective for treating bipolar depression than others?

Most of the research surrounding antidepressants refers almost exclusively to unipolar depression. There is no conclusive evidence that one antidepressant is more effective than another for treating bipolar depression. However, in a few controlled studies, researchers found that antidepressants worked better on bipolar depression than did lithium. Tegretol, in addition to its antimanic and prophylactic capabilities, does seem to have at least mild antidepressant effects. However, lithium and Depakote taken together with antidepressants do produce positive responses in most bipolar patients.

Which bipolar patients are most likely to swing from depression to mania while taking antidepressants?

According to many reports, bipolar I patients are most vulnerable to a drug-induced manic episode. Manic switches often occur in patients treated with tricyclics or MAOIs within a week of the first dose. A collaborative study by the Veterans Administration (VA) and the National Institute of Mental Health (NIMH) compared patients on both maintenance lithium and the tricyclic imipramine. The study, which included both unipolar and bipolar I patients, found that 67 percent of the bipolar patients on imipramine developed mania.

The few studies of bipolar depressed patients treated with MAOIs indicate a high rate of drug-induced mania. Three different studies, respectively, found 50 percent, 41 percent, and 35 percent of their subjects developing mania after short periods of time on MAOIs.

Some experts feel that the occurrence of switching for certain patients may be related to the natural course of their illness. Patients who have sequences of DMI (depression, which switches to mania or hypomania, and is then followed by an interval of wellness) may be more prone to antidepressant-induced swings. Those patients with the MDI sequence (mania, depression, interval of wellness) appear less susceptible.

Do antidepressants contribute to rapid cycling in depressed bipolar patients?

In some cases, yes. It appears that over the long-term course of the illness, antidepressants have the capacity to induce rapid cycling in some people. For patients whose illness is inherently more cyclical, antidepressants can increase the frequency and number of episodes. Antidepressant treatments can accelerate the rate of recovery, but they can also speed up the onset of the next episode. Patients can experience rapid cycling with both the continuous and intermittent use of antidepressants. Based on preliminary reports, experts believe that women are at a greater risk than men for antidepressant-induced rapid cycling. A history of mania and hypothyroidism also appears to be associated with drug-induced rapid cycling states.

What medications do doctors use for treating mixed and rapid cycling states?

Doctors initially place patients in mixed or rapid cycling states on a mood stabilizer. Formerly, doctors treated patients in these states with one drug, but now they generally use three or four medications at once. Depakote appears to be more effective than lithium for preventing the relapse of episodes. Combined, Depakote and lithium may work even better. Unfortunately, using the two medications together increases the possibility of side effects. Some clinicians administer Depakote, followed by Tegretol, and then a combination of Tegretol and lithium for optimal results.

Both Lamictal and Neurontin, anticonvulsants that are relatively new in the treatment of bipolar disorder, show great promise for patients who are severely depressed and experience rapid cycling. As we mentioned previously, calcium channel blockers may also prevent rapid cycling by limiting an excessive influx of calcium into brain cells. The calcium channel blocker Nimotop is particularly effective when combined with Tegretol.

One small study involved adding the stimulants

Ritalin or Dexedrine to standard bipolar medications. These drugs, most commonly used for treating attention deficit hyperactivity disorder (ADHD), seemed to reduce racing thoughts, irritability, and grandiose thoughts in most patients. They were not, however, found to be effective in limiting psychotic thinking.

What if the treatment for a mixed or rapid cycling patient is not fully effective and depression persists?

In these cases, clinicians should consider carefully administering an antidepressant. However, because research and clinical experience show that antidepressant use can aggravate mixed episodes and rapid cycling states, clinicians must exercise great caution. Closely monitoring a patient's condition and gathering information from family and friends about any new or different symptoms is crucial at this time.

Why would my doctor want to put me on maintenance medication?

Generally, bipolar patients suffer relapses of symptoms after acute symptoms of an episode have disappeared. It is the nature of bipolar disorder to be recurrent and for episodes to worsen and become more frequent as time goes by. Maintenance medication will, ideally, lessen the severity, frequency, and number of episodes over the course of the illness.

Lithium and Depakote are the primary medications used by clinicians for maintenance therapy. Tegretol and others, however, are now showing signs of promise for maintenance without some of the long-term effects of lithium. Experts have found lithium to be most effective when started as early as possible in patients.

According to a surfeit of data, lithium can greatly reduce both depressive and manic episodes, particularly in bipolar II patients. For those patients who stay on their maintenance medication, survival rate is comparable to that of the general population. Unfortunately, bipolar sufferers who go off their medication have a much shorter life expectancy.

What will happen if I stop taking my lithium?

Tragically, those patients who stop taking lithium after successful treatment may find the medication ineffective if they suffer a relapse. This is particularly true if an extensive amount of time has elapsed between the withdrawal from lithium and the onset of an episode. In addition, research indicates that patients who stop taking their lithium and then start again have a significantly higher rate of readmittance to psychiatric hospitals than do those who kept taking their medications. For patients who no longer respond to lithium, clinicians find that a combination of medications, such as lithium with Risperdal, is effective.

Will I still suffer episodes of mania and depression even if I comply with my maintenance medication?

Unfortunately, the answer is probably yes. When you have a relapse on medication it is called a "breakthrough" episode. Researchers are trying to uncover which medications, if any, can help prevent breakthrough episodes. Preliminary reports from one small study indicated that some patients on maintenance therapy found that Risperdal helped prevent breakthrough episodes of both mania and depression.

For those patients who do not respond to maintenance medication, maintenance ECT is showing some promise.

Will my doctor put me on maintenance medications right after I show the first signs of bipolar disorder?

You and your doctor will ultimately decide if and when you should begin taking maintenance medications. Generally, the principal selection criterion is a history of at least two major episodes. There are many considerations to take into account, including your overall tolerance to the medication, how well you respond to it, and if you are taking the medication on a regular basis. Most often, the decision to use maintenance medications comes after a patient has already been treated for an acute episode of mania or depression.

Despite the fact that most bipolar patients have enough recurrent episodes to warrant maintenance medication, not all patients receive prophylactic treatment right away. The doctor must consider the patient's age and gender as well as the type of episode, frequency, total number, and severity of prior episodes before making any decisions.

There is no question that bipolar patients who need hospitalization every year or two should be on some kind of maintenance regimen. Some studies have shown that patients who are frequently in the hospital have an average relapse rate of nearly 73 percent within the first year of diagnosis. Studies investigating the benefits of maintenance medication for patients with a lower relapse rate have yielded ambiguous results.

The truth is that every clinician handles maintenance and its attendant medications differently. Because of the irregular nature of the illness, some base their selection on the number rather than the frequency of episodes. Others feel that maintenance medication, after an initial episode of mania, is necessary for preventing the greatest number of potential future episodes.

What are some things my doctor will consider about my personality before prescribing maintenance medications?

Your doctor will consider several factors before placing you on maintenance medications, including:

- How reliable is the patient in detecting early signs of symptoms and in seeking treatment for these early warnings?
- Will the patient deny that anything is wrong until the

onset of a full-blown episode of mania or depression?

- What is the risk that the patient will attempt suicide?
- Does the patient have suitable family and psychiatric support systems in place?
- Will the patient's family be able to detect signs of hypomania?
- How has the patient responded in the past to the social and emotional burdens of taking maintenance medications?
- Is paying for medications an issue for the patient?
- Is the patient optimistic about recovery and treatment?

Additionally, the doctor must take into account how the patient handles stressful life events, how much stress currently exists in the patient's life, whether or not there is any physical illness, and the existence of alcohol or drug abuse.

Will my initial episode affect my maintenance medication?

If your initial bipolar episode is manic, maintenance medication is crucial. There is some evidence that if your initial bipolar episode is manic, you may be more susceptible to mania over the course of your illness. Early preventive treatment of subsequent episodes may lessen the frequency and severity of future ones. Therefore, most experts recommend prophylactic treatment for anyone who presents with mania. Because men appear to have a higher ratio of manic to depressive episodes than do women, men should begin maintenance medication as early as possible.

Compelling evidence suggests that the latency period between a first and second episode is longer in patients who have an early onset of bipolar disorder. Therefore, women between twenty-five and their early thirties may be able to postpone taking lithium and other mood stabilizers during their prime childbearing years. However, a doctor may determine that a patient is too unstable to delay prescribing them medication. Women who develop bipolar disorder before having children must address several important issues, including the inheritability of the illness and the potential for mood stabilizers to cause birth defects.

How long will I stay on maintenance medication after a manic episode?

After your first manic episode, you will probably take a maintenance medication for anywhere from six months to a year, or longer, depending on your response and symptoms. After you have had a second episode of mania, your doctor will recommend that you take maintenance medication for an indefinite period of time. However, you and your doctor will always reevaluate your condition. There is certainly the potential for readjusting your dosage to smaller amounts if your doctor feels it is safe to do so.

What are some of the side effects of long-term use of lithium?

Patients often stop taking their medications because they are concerned about side effects. If you have any questions, you should always talk to your doctor before you ever alter your plan or stop taking medication. Your doctor can always modify a dose or try a different drug if you have complaints about side effects.

The side effects of long-term lithium use include:

- Lithium toxicity (monitor levels frequently and alert patient to warning signs of central nervous system malfunctioning)
- Weight gain (frequently associated with poor compliance, can be managed by strict diet and exercise)
- A fine tremor (generally not difficult to treat)

- Polyuria or excessive urination (a diuretic can be used)
- Direct kidney damage (data is inconclusive)
- Lower thyroid functioning (doctor can administer a thyroid hormone)
- Sleep pattern disruption (can have a sedative or stimulant effect)

Most patients prefer to take as few doses of lithium a day as possible and to take them at night. When patients take high doses at night, the worst side effects tend to occur while they are sleeping, and thus they are generally unaware of them. Each individual requires different amounts of medication, and some may have to take more than one dose each day.

Why are "holidays" from maintenance medications not a good idea?

Certain experts recommend that patients have periods of time when they are not taking maintenance medications. Some clinicians take patients off medications because the patients need surgery or they are pregnant. These "holidays" generally allow the patient to both psychologically and physically heal from sustained use of the drugs. However, there are several downsides to taking a break from maintenance medications. It can take months to build up blood levels of certain drugs sufficient for them to be effective. Trying to achieve optimal blood levels again may be far more difficult than if you had just kept taking the medications in the first place.

Additionally, holidays may contribute to poor compliance. If the patient feels healthy off his medication for a certain period of time, he may think he no longer needs to take it. Clinicians should always decrease doses gradually and frequently check blood levels. Some patients feel more vulnerable during different times of the year and may have to have their lithium levels adjusted accordingly.

How do experts know if lithium is not working?

The three most obvious factors are:

1. Rapid cycling
2. Mixed manic and depressive states
3. Ongoing alcohol and drug abuse

Often the three conditions overlap and the patient has very poor compliance with prescribed treatment. Clinicians should immediately investigate new options, always trying to include patients as much as possible in the process.

Are there any alternatives to lithium for maintenance medications?

More and more, experts are finding that the anticonvulsants, like Depakote and Tegretol, are effective for maintenance use. Often, a clinician will use the drugs in combinations, depending on individual needs, their combined effectiveness, and the patient's tolerance.

Depakote is FDA approved and is emerging as a front-line maintenance medication along with lithium. Side effects appear to be few and quite mild. For maintenance, doctors administer a low dose initially, which they then gradually increase.

Next in line is Tegretol for maintenance therapy. Unfortunately, one emerging problem is that some patients relapse after successfully using Tegretol for many years. Side effects tend to be mild, but they may include:

1. Dizziness
2. Skin problems (e.g., acne)
3. Nausea and diarrhea
4. Drowsiness

5. Visual problems (e.g., blurred vision)
6. Slurred speech
7. Tremor
8. Confusion

How can combining different medications help bipolar patients who are "refractory," or resistant, to other forms of treatment?

Combining medications for medical conditions is a common practice. Clinicians use combination therapy to battle AIDS, congestive heart failure, and many different types of cancer. The authors of *The Role of Complex Combination Therapy in the Treatment of Refractory Bipolar Illness* (CNS Spectrums, 1998) believe that "it may also be rationalized that treating the patient with multiple agents that have different mechanisms of action may be associated with less toxicity and a better or more persistent therapeutic effect." In addition, by combining medications, clinicians are in most cases better able to control side effects.

Other factors that present a strong case for complex combination therapy for bipolar disorder are:

1. Clinicians from small and large hospitals and academic research centers report that an increasing number of patients are not responsive to medications used alone or in simple combinations. Patient need is the primary motivation for greater understanding and testing with complex combination drug therapies.

2. Recent studies indicate that 50 to 75 percent of patients tested did not respond to lithium monotherapy. Researchers also found that patients had no better response rate when the therapy included antidepressants for breakthrough depression and neuroleptics for breakthrough mania.

3. Investigators have found that when they add new agents, like Depakote and Tegretol, to the regimen, the patient's condition tends to improve dramatically.

How will my doctor determine whether using a combination of medications is best for me?

With so many new medications available, researchers and clinicians have had a great deal of difficulty determining the efficacy of all of the proposed medication combinations. There are a number of practical approaches that patients, their doctors, and their families can use to determine individual needs.

The recommendations are as follows:

1. Patients and their families should compile a detailed history of prior responses and reactions to medications. This helps clinicians explore what combinations the patient may now respond to.
2. Keeping a life chart of all past episodes, responses to medications, and when they took place is very useful for patients and their doctors. We will detail how to keep a life chart in chapter 8.
3. Patients should examine if there are any specific symptoms that remain unresponsive to medications. For example, a doctor may use a mood stabilizer with a more sedative effect for a patient who continues to have profound sleep disturbances.
4. Patients and their doctors need to assess which side effects are the most disruptive and choose the medications that are least problematic for them. In other words, two agents may essentially perform the same function, but one may cause fewer side effects in a particular patient.

Many more clinical trials need to be done before complex combination therapy becomes a standard for bipolar patients. In the future, clinicians may well be able to tailor an individual's medication treatment to his or her own specific biology, psychology, and history.

Is medication my only choice?

The reality for most individuals with bipolar disorder is that medication is and will remain their first form of treatment. Fortunately, medications for bipolar disorder are constantly being refined and are becoming less and less disruptive to those dependent on them. Patients and doctors should realize that each individual responds to medications in subtle and different ways. The use of medications is a thoughtful clinical art applied to science by a skilled, experienced, and concerned psychiatrist.

Medications do not have to define you or your illness, but you do have to take them to remain healthy. There are a number of other treatment options for bipolar patients, but most are adjunctive to medication. In chapter 7 we will present some of the more compelling alternative treatments available for those looking to explore new possibilities in managing the disorder.

Chapter 7

OTHER THERAPIES FOR BIPOLAR DISORDER

Are medication and psychotherapy the only treatments available to help people with bipolar disorder?

Drug therapy is almost always the primary treatment for bipolar patients. Psychotherapy enhances medication treatments, adding greater fulfillment and stability to the lives of those with the disorder. Currently, the only other clinically approved alternative to medication treatment is electroconvulsive therapy, or ECT. For those people who spend extended periods as inpatients, hospitals provide several types of therapy to help make the transition back into mainstream society easier. These include recreational, vocational, and group therapies.

Bipolar patients must take special care when investigating other available therapies like phototherapy and hypnotherapy, because these treatments may precipitate mania and increase paranoia. Whether exploring the effects of sleep deprivation or engaging in self-help activities like meditation and visualization, you must always exercise caution. Informing your doctor and your family of any changes in your therapy regimen or daily activities can prevent minor fluctuations in behavior from escalating into full-blown episodes.

ELECTROCONVULSIVE THERAPY (ECT)

What is electroconvulsive therapy?

Since its introduction in the 1930s, ECT or "shock treatment" has been much maligned. Mention ECT to most people and images of patients violently restrained against their will, wires attached to their heads, and wildly convulsing tend to come to mind. And while doctors often misused ECT in its early stages, the procedure has been consistently refined over the last sixty years. Many clinicians now find ECT an extremely useful tool and commonly employ the technique for treating both bipolar manic and depressed patients.

The procedure begins with the administration of a muscle relaxant and a short-acting anesthetic. Next, a physician attaches either one or two electrodes to a patient's temple(s) and then sends a high-voltage current into and through the brain. This current causes a generalized seizure or convulsion that lasts about forty seconds. The seizures alter brain chemistry and can temporarily relieve both manic and depressive symptoms. It is not easy to observe the seizure because of the patient's relaxed muscles, so doctors track its progression on an electroencephalogram monitor (EEG).

Studies have shown that ECT affects the same neurotransmitters as do many of the antidepressants discussed in chapter 6. Additionally, the procedure stimulates the endorphin system, which releases hormones that act as natural opiates. These hormones are generally responsible for elevating a patient's mood, but the specific mechanism is still unknown.

Why would my doctor choose ECT over medication?

There are several reasons why doctors might choose ECT over medication. Some experts even believe that ECT may be more effective than certain medications for treating severely manic patients. One review of studies showed that 470 out of 589 patients (80 percent) who were treated with ECT for acute mania showed significant clinical improvement.

Reasons for choosing ECT include:

1. When the patient is unresponsive to prescribed medications
2. When the patient is pregnant and unable to take mood stabilizers because of the risk of birth defects
3. Patients who have specific heart conditions that preclude the use of certain bipolar medications
4. Those patients in mixed states with a high risk of suicide
5. Occasionally when the patient has a rare syndrome of manic delirium (may be associated with severe hyperthermia)
6. If the patient has other medical conditions that preclude the use of the bipolar medications
7. For patients with psychotic depression who are unresponsive to medication

Treatment decisions are always subject to reevaluation by patients and their doctors. Some patients take medication for a while, then use ECT, then go back on medication when and if necessary. Generally, experts do not recommend that patients use ECT *while* taking medication because of possible adverse interactions. However, there are exceptions, which we will discuss later in this chapter.

How will the physician control the amount of electrical charge going through my brain?

Experts have refined ECT equipment over the past several decades. With carefully calibrated machines and monitors, technicians are now able to precisely control the amount of electricity passing into and through the brain. Once the procedure is finished, you will continue to be monitored by your doctor so she can evaluate both the effects and possible side effects of ECT.

Does ECT cause any side effects?

Yes. Though generally mild and not terribly disruptive, you may experience:

1. Temporary confusion
2. Memory lapses
3. Headaches
4. Nausea
5. Muscle soreness
6. Heart disturbances

Compared to the side effects that patients can experience while taking medication, ECT side effects tend to be fewer and last a much shorter time.

I've heard that ECT can cause memory loss. Is this true?

Yes, but the loss is usually only temporary. Some evidence shows that placing electrodes unilaterally and on the patient's nondominant side greatly reduces the risk of any memory dysfunction. Studies show that the patient's capacity to retain, learn, and recall new information is undisturbed six to nine months after treatment.

The most acute memory loss takes place about thirty minutes after an ECT treatment, when patients regain consciousness. Short-term memory suffers the most, with patients unable to recall events leading up to and following the session. In addition to having difficulty with names, addresses, dates, and phone numbers, patients have no memory of the actual ECT session. As mentioned above, most patients regain what they have lost after a few months. However, a few patients complain of continued memory loss years after treatment. Occasionally, a patient suffers permanent damage (e.g., an inability to learn new information and recall old information) after receiving bilateral ECT. The general advantage of bilateral over unilateral ECT, however, is fewer required treatments.

Possible memory loss should not discourage patients

from exploring the use of ECT. Patients need to learn as much as they can about ECT and then weigh the benefits and risks. Both research and clinical studies have shown the treatment to be quite effective for bipolar patients. It is encouraging that the great majority of patients who have been treated with ECT do not suffer significant or long-lasting memory loss.

Would a doctor ever recommend bilateral electrode placement over unilateral?

It depends on the case. If a doctor feels that bilateral placement would be more effective for a particular patient than unilateral, then he might recommend it. Some experts feel that to obtain the full antimanic effects of ECT, electrodes should be placed on both temples. There is no definitive data suggesting that bilateral placement has greater effectiveness, and doctors should use their experience and discretion to decide what is best for the patient.

How does ECT work in the brain?

ECT uses electrical charges to change brain chemistry. Despite extensive research, experts still do not completely understand how the procedure alters chemicals in the brain. Somehow, convulsions (electrically induced repetitive firing of neurons) modify the brain's chemical messenger systems. The action is somewhat analogous to cardio-conversion, which electrically restores the heart to a normal rhythm. However, cardio-conversion uses far more electricity than ECT.

Can doctors use ECT for maintenance purposes?

A number of studies have found ECT to be helpful for those patients who do not respond to or cannot tolerate a regimen of maintenance medication. Researchers in one study chose bipolar patients for possible ECT maintenance who had recurrent episodes that were unresponsive to medication treatment. Clinicians ordered monthly ECT treatments for the subjects that lasted for more than a year and a half. Before the treatments, the patients suffered, on average, at least three episodes annually and spent almost half a year in the hospital. After the ECT treatments, all of the rapid-cycling patients in the study experienced full or partial remission of symptoms.

How many ECT sessions will I need?

For unipolar depression, experts usually recommend a course of six to twelve ECT treatments administered two to three times per week. Individual patients may need fewer or more sessions, depending on their response to ECT. Several studies that compare rates of ECT response between unipolar and bipolar depressed patients show that the treatment is equally effective for both disorders. The number and frequency of sessions for unipolar and bipolar depression is generally the same. As a result, ECT is considered extremely effective for treating bipolar depression.

The general recommendation for manic patients is three ECT treatments per week. Manic patients usually respond quite rapidly to treatments, but there appears to be no difference in response rates (i.e., no added benefit) with more frequent treatments than three times per week. Patients can show a complete remission in as few as six treatments, but the number tends to vary depending on the individual. The doctor, ideally with the help of the patient, will reassess the patient's condition and the effects of the treatment after each session.

Who is in the room with the patient during an ECT treatment?

A team of people is in the room with a patient receiving ECT. This team usually includes a psychiatrist, an anesthesiologist, and a psychiatric nurse working together to administer the treatment.

Can ECT provoke a hypomanic or manic episode?

Yes, but this is rare. As a result, there are still no specific guidelines for practitioners when it does happen. Some doctors discontinue the use of ECT and begin administering a mood stabilizer. Other practitioners carry on with ECT treatments.

Can I take any other bipolar medications during ECT treatments?

Yes, but doctors must take great care to try to minimize adverse interactions. Doctors who give patients lithium during ECT may be putting them at a higher risk for delirium and epilepsy. These reactions, however, are quite rare. If symptoms persist, doctors should take patients off lithium. Doctors generally do not recommend using anticonvulsants, such as Depakote and Tegretol, with ECT, as the medications can interfere with the ECT process. These reactions are very complex, and more research needs to be done to determine how ECT and bipolar medications interact.

Benzodiazepines (e.g., Klonopin and Ativan) tend to raise a person's seizure threshold and reduce the duration and intensity of seizures. Their effects may interfere with the efficacy of ECT and render the treatment virtually useless. Antipsychotic medications (e.g., Haldol and Thorazine) can be used during the course of ECT for those patients who are highly agitated and psychotic. Once the symptoms abate, however, doctors usually stop using antipsychotics.

What is the cost of an ECT session?

Single sessions of ECT generally run from $650 to $1,000, depending on where the treatment is being done and who is administering it. The fee covers the use of the ECT suite, which is usually a surgical facility at a hospital. In addition, it includes the ECT equipment, medication, and the fees for the anesthesiologist and psychiatrist. Every insurance company and HMO has a different policy regarding the percentage of each session and how many sessions they will cover. Generally, insurance will cover ECT for most patients.

Do any contraindications exist for ECT?

Experts are not aware of any absolute contraindications to ECT. However, doctors generally recommend that people with cardiovascular disease or brain lesions, which can include tumors that put pressure on the brain, not use ECT.

I'm a little nervous about the idea of ECT. What can help me overcome my fears?

Learning more about an unknown quantity—in this case a treatment and procedure—is often the best way to allay your fears of it. ECT is not for everyone, but for many patients it is the safest and most effective treatment for bipolar disorder. Unfortunately, it is underutilized because past stigmas about ECT persist. Asking your doctor or another clinician about the procedure and having her detail what will happen, the effects, and the possible side effects, is a good place to start. Support groups and group therapy are excellent forums for discussing your apprehensions and meeting others who have undergone the treatment.

According to the 1985 National Institutes Statement on ECT, patients have varied experiences regarding the procedure. Several patients found the experience terrifying, invasive, and shameful to talk about with those unfamiliar with the treatment. Some reported persistent memory loss, while still others found ECT to be a wholly beneficial and even lifesaving necessity.

As with almost any treatment, no two patients will react to ECT the same way. Understanding as much as you can about the procedure and the course of your own condition will help you come to a decision. Remember, you are not alone with your fears, and you should always feel free to seek support for these and other important issues.

HOSPITALIZATION

Do all bipolar patients spend time in hospitals?

No. In fact, many patients never have to spend even one night in a hospital because of their bipolar disorder. Bipolar disorder is an illness that doctors can treat on a continual outpatient basis except in the most severe cases. Hospitalization may be necessary, but with close attention to symptoms, careful monitoring from both physicians and family, medication compliance, and psychotherapeutic support, it should be the exception, not the rule.

Why are patients admitted to the hospital?

Hospitalization may be necessary for those patients who are acutely suicidal, homicidal, psychotic, or highly agitated (if the patient has the potential for becoming more dangerous). Additionally, if a doctor deems a patient's medical health particularly poor, then she may suggest a stay in the hospital. Professionals do not casually admit bipolar patients into the hospital. There are also several legal and practical steps that doctors and family members must first take, some of which we have discussed in chapter 5.

Individuals receive treatment as inpatients at both public and private hospitals. General hospitals also have psychiatric units specifically designed to treat those patients with mental illnesses. In the hospital, patients tend to receive treatment from a team of professionals, not just their psychiatrist. These team members can include residents, psychologists, social workers, psychiatric nurses, occupational therapists, vocational therapists, and recreational therapists.

Ideally, each member of the team contributes to better your well-being and expedite your release from the hospital.

What happens to bipolar patients once they have been admitted to the hospital?

After a complete physical examination, including blood tests and an electrocardiogram (EKG), a doctor will stabilize you on medication or administer ECT if necessary. Once you are stabilized, the doctor will make further physical and psychological assessments regarding your condition. He may elicit help from your family doctor, other psychiatrists, psychologists, and family members. From these results, he will determine how long he wants you to stay as an inpatient. He will continue to reevaluate your condition, with the help of other team members, on a daily basis.

Like patients in the hospital for surgical (invasive) or voluntary (cosmetic) procedures, you will sleep in a private or semiprivate room. You will eat meals in a dining room with other patients and wear street clothes instead of hospital gowns. Generally, the staff will also wear street clothes, but this can vary from facility to facility. Most hospitals have recreational and leisure areas where patients can play games, watch television, or engage in art projects.

Will I start psychotherapy in the hospital?

A large portion of your time in the hospital will be spent learning to cope with your illness. Your psychiatric team will primarily concentrate on psychoeducation, teaching you and your family about how to manage and live with bipolar disorder. You will probably have a number of daily therapy sessions, ranging from cognitive-behavioral therapy to recreational therapy. Some sessions will be individual or with your immediate family, while others will include a group of patients from the hospital. Group and communal activities probably will include patients with a number of different conditions other than bipolar disorder. Hospitals tend to mix their patients together rather than separate them based on illness. Obviously, if a patient is psychotic or poses a threat, he will be separated from other patients until he is stabilized.

Psychotherapy sessions take place on average about

three to five times a week. They are generally shorter than the "fifty-minute hour," because many patients are agitated or cannot concentrate for long periods of time. Your individual sessions may be run by your admitting psychiatrist or another staff doctor. Your other therapeutic sessions will be conducted by staff psychiatrists, supervised psychiatric residents, clinical social workers, occupational therapists, and recreational therapists. If you are receiving ECT, clinicians will schedule your psychotherapeutic appointments around the treatments.

Can talking to other patients help me to feel better?

You may find it very therapeutic to share with other patients experiences about your illness, your impressions of the hospital, and your fears about being released. Being exposed to "milieu therapy" (the idea that the psychiatric unit of a hospital can itself be therapeutic) is beneficial for many inpatients. You may even find that you are less inhibited discussing your feelings with other patients than with your various therapists. Encounters with other patients generally occur during unstructured activities, such as meal and leisure times. Group therapy sessions are also excellent settings to securely exchange ideas with other patients. Community meetings give patients a sense of empowerment by giving them a forum to discuss hospital politics, services, and the overall environment.

For many people, just knowing they are not alone is a substantial benefit derived from sharing with fellow patients.

What are some of the therapies psychiatric hospitals offer?

The services that a psychiatric hospital offers depends quite a bit on its philosophy and budget. If hospital administrators think patients will benefit from involvement in activities that reinforce their self-esteem and give them a sense of purpose, they will probably try to provide a number of therapeutic options. The services a hospital is able to provide are often in direct proportion to its operating budget. A well-funded private hospital may have more special services for patients than its large, underfunded public counterpart.

Some of the therapies hospital staff provide are:

• *Group therapy:* As we discussed in chapter 5, group therapy is an excellent place for patients to exchange ideas and share experiences common to those with mental illnesses. Hospital sessions usually consist of six to ten patients and one or two professionals. Serving as group leaders, these psychiatrists, psychologists, or clinical social workers facilitate open communication in a secure setting. Sessions often revolve around a theme (e.g., depression, coping with symptoms) and patients tend to do the bulk of the talking. Changing destructive behaviors and coping skills are two central goals of group therapy.

• *Recreational therapy:* Led by a recreational therapist or "therapeutic recreation worker," this type of therapy consists of medically approved recreation activities for inpatients. The activities include: sports, dramatics, games, and arts and crafts. The goals of recreational therapy are for patients to socialize with greater ease, establish healthy interpersonal relationships, become confident participating in a group, and have fun.

• *Vocational therapy:* Admission to a hospital is often very disruptive to a person's academic or professional life. Patients must learn skills and develop a plan for returning to the pressures and responsibilities of school or work. Vocational therapists help patients discover their interests and develop their professional abilities in a safe and secure setting. Reentering the workforce or going back to school can be very daunting to patients just out of the hospital. Ideally, vocational therapy helps patients ease back into the workplace and, by extension, everyday life outside the hospital.

• *Occupational therapy:* Before patients arrive at the hospital, they usually have had a hard time taking care of themselves. Just making breakfast, getting dressed, and cleaning the house can seem like overwhelming tasks. Occupational therapy aims to teach patients how to perform simple daily tasks that might otherwise appear daunting. Most occupational therapists work with physically handicapped individuals who need help with the most basic functions. However, many mentally ill patients reap great benefits from someone helping them organize a schedule and create a plan for self-sufficiency.

How long will I stay in the hospital?

That depends on the severity of your condition, on when your doctor feels ready to release you, and insurance company and HMO constraints. Most depressed patients stay in the hospital for about two weeks. Over the past fifteen years or so, hospital stays have generally decreased owing to cuts in funding for public facilities, third-party payment, and managed care. Furthermore, lengths of stay are shorter because patients have received better overall care.

If your doctor feels you are still at risk for suicide or if you are still in a highly unstable condition, he will recommend that you continue treatment in the hospital. Most doctors, however, are able to continue treating bipolar patients on an outpatient basis after a few weeks in the hospital. Ideally, bipolar patients go from the psychiatric hospital environment to a supportive and informed family one.

How much will it cost me to be in a psychiatric facility?

Costs for inpatient care vary from hospital to hospital. It is not unheard of for some facilities to charge over $1,000 a day. Your insurance company or HMO will pay a portion of the expense. Make sure you or a family member asks your provider how many days and what percentage will be covered in the hospital.

How do I know if I'm in a good hospital?

Hopefully your family will be your advocate if you are unable to speak for yourself about the psychiatric facility. Some people believe they will receive better care at a private hospital than a public one, but this is not always the case. Two helpful indicators of a hospital's quality are recommendations from former patients and doctors you trust and whether the hospital is affiliated with a good medical school. Additionally, the experience of the staff and the number that are board certified often directly correlate to the level of care you receive.

If you have recently been diagnosed with bipolar disorder, it is not imprudent to do a check of some of the better psychiatric facilities in the country. It may seem like an odd task, but it might prove useful someday. According to *U.S. News & World Report* (1998), a few of the top-ranked psychiatric facilities in the United States are:

1. Massachusetts General Hospital (Boston, Massachusetts)

2. C. F. Menninger Memorial Hospital (Topeka, Kansas)

3. McLean Hospital (Belmont, Massachusetts)

4. Johns Hopkins Hospital (Baltimore, Maryland)

5. New York Hospital–Cornell Medical Center (New York, New York)

6. The Mayo Clinic (Rochester, Minnesota)

7. UCLA Neuropsychiatric Hospital (Los Angeles, California)

8. Columbia-Presbyterian Medical Center (New York, New York)

9. Sheppard and Enoch Pratt Hospital (Baltimore, Maryland)

10. Yale–New Haven Hospital (New Haven, Connecticut)

The magazine ranked the hospitals according to their reputations among some of the country's leading psychiatrists.

REPETITIVE TRANSCRANIAL MAGNETIC STIMULATION (rTMS)

What is repetitive transcranial magnetic stimulation?

A new procedure, rTMS entails applying a magnetic force to the surface of the brain. ECT sends a high-voltage current that jolts the entire brain. Repetitive transcranial magnetic stimulation trains a high-voltage current directly on the problem area of the brain, in this case the prefrontal cortex. As with ECT, the exact mechanism of rTMS is unknown, but somehow it enhances the efficacy of neurotransmitters in the mood centers of the brain. Because there is no need to anesthetize the patient and there are no convulsions (although they can occur as a side effect), rTMS appears to be safer and less invasive than ECT. Also, there is the possibility of no memory loss.

Dr. Martin Szuba, a psychiatrist at the University of Pennsylvania, administered rTMS to twelve patients who found no relief from depression with either medication or ECT. After two weeks of daily twenty-minute treatments, seven of the twelve patients showed moderate to dramatic results. The effects lasted for up to a month before the patients needed more rTMS sessions.

Some experts believe that the procedure may someday replace ECT for treating both depression and mania. Most of the ongoing clinical studies—some twenty trials—involve only depression. Currently, both New York University School of Medicine and the National Institute of Mental Health (NIMH), among others, are conducting rigorous studies.

How do doctors administer repetitive transcranial magnetic stimulation?

The doctor uses an electromagnetic coil held against the scalp to pass the pulses of high-voltage current into the brain. The coil is shaped and positioned relative to the scalp, so the stimulation on the brain tissue can be quite specific and localized. The current generates a rapidly alternating magnetic field, creating an electric current that can depolarize neutral brain tissue.

Before rTMS replaces ECT for treatment of depression and mania, researchers must determine the optimal wave form, frequency, and amplitude for provoking seizures.

Can omega-3 fatty acids help in the treatment of bipolar disorder?

Possibly. Omega-3 fatty acids are a class of polyunsaturated lipids found in fish oil. In one study, conducted at Harvard Medical School, the acids seemed to be helpful in a number of cases. The four-month study compared the efficacy of high doses of omega-3 fatty acids (about nine grams a day) versus a placebo amount of olive oil. All of the patients in the study had unstable bipolar disorder.

Only *one* of fifteen patients who received omega-3 fatty acids suffered a recurrence of symptoms during the period that researchers studied them. Interestingly, seven of fifteen patients who took the placebo reported a recurrence of symptoms. The only adverse effect of the omega-3 fatty acids that patients reported was mild, dose-related gastrointestinal distress. The authors speculated that the fish oil may decrease the overfiring of nerve cells in the mood centers of the brain, similar to one mechanism proposed for lithium and Depakote.

At least in this initial study, it does appear that omega-3 fatty acids may have a mood-stabilizing effect in patients with unstable bipolar disorder. Researchers need to repeat the omega-3 tests with larger numbers of patients over a longer period of time.

Should I take herbal remedies or hormones for depression if I have bipolar disorder?

Not unless you have thoroughly discussed doing so with your doctor. In recent years, several herbal remedies and hormones for treating depression have appeared on the market, including St. John's wort *(hypericum perforatum)* and melatonin. These substances may have positive effects for depression, but there is no understanding of how they affect mania or bipolar disorder in general. One meta-analysis of St. John's wort involved twenty-three studies and more than 1,700 outpatients. Researchers came to the conclusion that extracts of St. John's wort appeared to have similar effects as standard antidepressants for treating mild to moderate unipolar depression. However, there have been no studies conducted to determine how St. John's wort affects bipolar patients and interacts with other drugs, and no studies done to determine its side effects.

People use the hormone melatonin most commonly for reducing or eliminating jet lag. Recently, there have been some indications that it may have mood-elevating properties when taken alone or with antidepressants. As of this writing, however, there have been no large-scale studies performed that prove melatonin's effectiveness or safety, especially for bipolar patients. The fact that melatonin is a hormone, and may potentially interact with other hormones in adverse ways, is of particular concern for bipolar patients.

Generally, people taking medication for bipolar disorder should avoid experimenting with substances that have not been proven to be clinically effective for the illness. Taking part in a controlled study of a new substance, such as omega-3 fatty acids, that has potential as a bipolar treatment usually means you are under the watchful eyes of experts. We can only hope that in the future the myriad of herbal and alternative substances currently flooding the market will be subject to the same rigorous testing standards as mainstream prescription medications are now.

How does sleep deprivation affect bipolar disorder?

Adjusting sleep patterns is one way clinicians are experimenting with treating bipolar patients. Since sleep disturbances are one of the first symptomatic indicators of a bipolar episode, understanding how alterations in sleep affect the patient may prove useful. Studies have shown that total sleep deprivation and partial sleep deprivation during the second half of the night (usually after two or three A.M.) can temporarily relieve unipolar and bipolar depression. Despite the fact that some patients suffer a relapse after sleeping again, a certain portion of patients report the ensuing depression to be less profound.

Unfortunately, any alteration in sleep patterns can also precipitate mania. Some experts advise patients that even one night of unexplainable sleep loss can be the early warning signs of an impending manic episode. Always talk to your doctor and inform your family if you are going to experiment with sleep deprivation to combat depression.

Can hypnotherapy have negative effects for bipolar patients?

Yes, and it is generally not recommended. Hypnosis is used psychotherapeutically (by therapists) to put patients in a relaxed state of wakefulness and a heightened condition of awareness and suggestibility. While hypnotized, the patient responds to appropriate questions from the hypnotherapist. In a hypnotic state, memories become more vivid, moods more intense, and perceptions highly acute. For bipolar patients, especially those prone to delusions, paranoia, and psychosis, hypnosis may increase the possibility of both manic and depressive symptoms. Memories of past traumas and realizations of perceived inadequacies can become too real for the bipolar patient.

Unless your doctor recommends hypnotherapy, it is probably safer for you to engage in therapies that keep you grounded in reality and focused on the present.

What is light therapy, and does it pose any risks for bipolar patients?

Doctors often suggest light therapy, or phototherapy, for patients who are suffering mild to severe depression. It is especially useful for those patients who suffer depression from light deprivation or seasonal affective disorder (SAD). For more information about SAD, consult *If You Think You Have Seasonal Affective Disorder,* also in the Dell Guides for Mental Health series. Light therapy involves exposing yourself to a wide-spectrum artificial light source for a period of between two and four hours each day.

Interestingly, the therapeutic effects from light therapy seem to relate directly to the eyes and not the skin. After years of accumulated experience, experts have found no adverse effects on the eyes of those patients who regularly use light therapy. Like sleep-deprivation therapy, light therapy acts rapidly and the action stops roughly when the treatment does.

With respect to bipolar disorder, light therapy may be most useful for bipolar II patients. This form of the disorder has a pattern similar to SAD, with an onset of depressive symptoms in the autumn and winter. Depressive symptoms then abate in the spring and a more hypomanic condition develops during the summer. Bipolar I patients are at some risk for developing manic symptoms with light therapy. If the light therapy causes significant swings in mood, disturbances in sleep function, or alterations in normal behavior patterns, you should probably discontinue treatment.

Are there any self-help techniques that might be useful for alleviating symptoms of bipolar disorder?

No matter which alternative treatments you decide to investigate, they should never interfere with your medication regimen. Discussing options with your doctor and informing your family are also of critical importance; these people may be the first to notice any changes in your mood or behavior. In addition to any self-help techniques you try, remember to maintain regular sleep patterns and avoid alcohol and caffeine.

You may want to explore any number of techniques that will improve your overall mood, mental state, and physical condition. These may include the following:

1. *Exercise:* It has long been known that routine, aerobic exercise increases levels of endorphins (hormones that lift mood) in the brain. Sustained, regular exercise, such as swimming, running, walking, and biking can relieve several forms of depression. Levels of serotonin and norepinephrine have been shown to increase in the brain after exercise. Both of these may relieve depressive symptoms and give you an overall sense of well-being. If you notice yourself inclined or driven to do more than your normal amount of daily or weekly exercise, hypomania may be incipient. Alert a family member or call your doctor to discuss other possibly nascent symptoms.

2. *Meditation:* Reducing stress and bringing one's mental, physical, and emotional self into balance are central principles of meditation. There are several forms of the technique, most having derived from Eastern philosophy and teachings. People generally meditate in a peaceful and quiet setting, either lying or sitting down. Other types of meditation are dynamic and involve dancing wildly to loud music. Ideally, meditation allows you to set aside a block of time during the day to focus on feeling better, healing yourself, and letting go of concerns that may be weighing heavily on you. Thoughts should drift in and out of your mind. Some practitioners encourage trying not to think of anything at all. Meditation alone is probably most beneficial for mild to moderate forms of depression. For a major depressive episode, meditation may be useful in conjunction with medication and psychotherapy. Many severely depressed people find it too difficult to establish the focus and concentration needed to meditate. Hypomanic and manic patients are generally unable to sit still long

enough to achieve a meditative state. Meditation can help patients who feel overstimulated to calm down. Removing yourself from a stressful situation by closing your eyes and trying not to think may prevent a mood swing.

3. *Visualization:* Patients with a variety of medical conditions from cancer to heart disease use visualization to alleviate stress and imagine themselves well. A therapist trained in the technique or well-produced audiotapes can help you achieve a peaceful and meditative state where you conjure images that make you feel empowered and healthy. A depressed patient may visualize a group of hands that boost him up a ladder to the next level in his life, giving him a sense of accomplishment and pride. Again, visualization is best used for depressed or euthymic patients, since many hypomanic and manic patients are unable to concentrate long enough or at all. The technique is not recommended for patients with a history or presence of delusions, hallucinations, paranoia, or psychotic behavior.

Can acupuncture be useful for bipolar patients?

The Chinese have used acupuncture for more than five thousand years to treat almost every known bodily ailment. This form of Chinese medicine uses very thin needles or needles with an electric current passed through them to stimulate specific points on the body. By restoring the normal flow of bioelectric energy, or "qi," acupuncture attempts to activate the body's own healing systems. The technique has been shown to relieve both mild and severe depression in some patients, with no apparent sign of side effects. For a more detailed look at acupuncture and its use against depression, refer to *If You Think You Have Depression* in the Dell Guides for Mental Health series.

With respect to acupuncture and its use in acute mania, there have been no significant studies. However, slipping hair-thin needles into a highly agitated and manic individual seems unrealistic at best. It would be interesting to see if acupuncture might work prophylactically against future manic episodes, but as of this writing there have been no studies in this area either.

Are there other ways for bipolar patients to cope with their illness?

Yes. In the final chapter of this book, we will look at ways that bipolar patients can learn to cope with this often chronic condition. Medication is a central element to effectively treating bipolar disorder, but you also need to develop ways to observe changes in your own mood and develop a set of life-managing skills. It is not always an easy or straightforward task, but establishing a low-stress and ordered life will add to greater feelings of control and happiness.

Chapter 8

COPING WITH BIPOLAR DISORDER

Why is it important for bipolar patients to maintain ongoing relationships with their doctors and therapists?

Each individual case of bipolar disorder is always changing. The illness continuously presents new emotional, physical, and psychological challenges for its patients. At certain points you may feel in complete control of your life. At other times, nothing seems right—not work, not family, not even your very existence. Coping with the vicissitudes of bipolar disorder is not a task you can easily handle alone, nor does anyone expect you to. Knowing that there are professionals who understand how quickly your outlook and moods can change is fundamental to navigating the inevitably difficult times.

There are several ways to make managing bipolar disorder a collaborative effort between not only you and your doctor, but also you and your family. Taking part in your own care by keeping mood charts, developing self-rating systems, and keeping abreast of the latest treatment developments is empowering and helps to build self-esteem. Establishing long-term relationships with one or a group of professionals allows them time to learn who you are and the nature of your illness. The comfort that comes from knowing that your doctor understands you can be immeasurable.

Why is it important for me to take a substantial role in my own care?

The more you take part in your own care, the greater the chances of leading a stable and productive life. When bipolar patients are severely depressed or manic, they tend to have little interest in caring for themselves. Thus it is often helpful to make plans for the future during the calmer, more neutral periods. Patients and their families should remain educated about bipolar disorder by watching films, reading books, attending lectures, and talking with professionals about new treatment developments.

With any luck, your doctor will have discussed the possibility of future hospitalizations with you and your family before the need should ever arise. When patients are rational, they may decide they want to use ECT or another treatment regimen for future depressive or manic episodes. Because people are unlikely to consent to the procedure in the midst of a severe episode, some states allow doctors and patients to draw up informed consent agreements. This enables the patient to consent to certain treatments before actually needing them. Before you sign any such agreements, make sure you speak to your attorney and the attorney at the hospital where the procedure would take place, and check with your local psychiatric association regarding the law in your state. By calling one of the national mental health organizations, you can obtain information about any federal legislation that pertains to informed consent.

Making anticipatory consents to treatments is not an easy or simple choice. Before a manic or depressive episode happens, patients should always spend some time considering their options and what is best for them.

How can I keep track of all the changes in my mood and treatment over long periods of time?

One of the most helpful ways is to keep a graph that charts mood and drug response changes over time. These charts provide invaluable information regarding:

- how seasonal and premenstrual patterns affect mood
- how psychological and biological changes correlate with mood swings
- responsiveness to treatment
- worsening of illness due to certain treatments (e.g., increased cycling due to use of antidepressants)
- compliance with medication
- number of mood swings over a certain period of time
- general course of the illness
- how stressful life events may precipitate bipolar episodes

Charting moods and other pertinent information also gives patients a sense of control and power when dealing with their illness. The charts provide patients with concrete proof that their treatment plan is (a) working and (b) may need modifying at certain points. Doctors may find it useful to share examples of other patients' mood charts (preserving these patients' anonymity, of course) with their patients to demonstrate different patterns of mood shifts. An essential teaching point of sharing mood charts is to illustrate to patients that recovery patterns can have an uneven and unpredictable course. This is true even when patients are carefully monitored. Using the charts to predict episode frequency and duration may help to minimize a patient's discouragement during challenging periods.

What are some specific examples of mood charts?

One example is a chart that graphs how mental states affect physical activity or psychomotor responses. Patients draw a time line across a piece of paper and a vertical line on the left side of the time line. They then write a range of numbers between −5 and +5. Minus five represents a severely depressive state, which would require admission to a hospital. At −5, the patient is unable to function normally, has lost her appetite, and lacks the energy to get out of bed in the morning. Moving up the scale from −5 toward 0, the depressive state abates.

Zero indicates a normal mood state and ability to function. As the numbers increase on the positive side, the patient becomes increasingly manic. Plus one is a slightly more energetic and active state than 0 (e.g., early signs of hypomania). Plus five is an acute manic episode, complete with an abundance of energy, disrupted sleep patterns, racing thoughts, and, in some instances, hospitalization.

Patients chart each day by making marks on the scale that indicate their psychomotor state. Then they connect that mark with the previous day's mark. Over time, the chart reflects how the day-to-day changes in physical activity correspond to mood alterations. Patients also factor any significant physical or emotional events that might affect mood states (e.g., menstruation, birth of a child, death of a parent, changes in medication dosage). Patients should always record any changes they deem relevant.

After tracking information for several months, patients and their doctors can then determine patterns that may be affecting treatment and normal functioning. If necessary, the doctor can modify medications or recommend that the patient pursue less stressful activities.

Patients often find it hard to be diligent about recording information on their charts. They should enlist the help of parents and spouses when they are unable to muster the energy, cannot remember, or lose interest in maintaining the chart themselves.

Is it useful to keep a life chart for children who show signs of bipolar disorder?

Many adult bipolar patients feel that using life charts helps them to control their illness. Similarly, charting the behavioral course of children who present bipolar symptoms, without actually meeting the full criteria for the illness, is a useful tracking and diagnostic tool. According to the *Bipolar Network News* (July 1997), "It is equally apparent that the early presentations of bipolar illness can be extremely diverse and pleomorphic, not necessarily displaying discrete periods of classic mania or depression." Thus when parents and doctors create a life chart for a child with a mood disturbance, they must include a greater range of behaviors. These may include tantrums, aggression toward others or self, and refusal to obey parents and teachers.

Charting a child's moods and behaviors at both home and school is extremely useful for early intervention and treatment of incipient bipolar disorder and other mood dysfunctions. The life chart should graph:

1. Degree of symptoms (low, mild, moderate, or high)
2. Family, social, and academic problems
3. Any medical interventions or hospitalizations
4. Inability to function at home or school
5. Number and duration of episodes
6. Type of episodes
7. Age when abnormal behavior began
8. Years, months, and days
9. Aggressive behavior
10. Tantrums
11. Alterations in sleep patterns

Children can become very self-conscious if their every move is charted. Putting a child under a behavioral "microscope" is probably unnecessary and may aggravate her condition rather than alleviate symptoms.

How can I learn to discriminate between a normal and abnormal mood?

Detecting when your mood is beginning to swing is a formidable but not impossible task. Patients who have lived with bipolar disorder for many years often become quite sensitive to their moods. Other patients who are not as aware of their moods may have to depend on their support network of family members and friends to help them, especially at first. If you live with your parents or a spouse, they will soon become, if they are not already, very aware of your mood shifts and behavioral changes. Patients who live alone may have a harder time finding someone to help detect alterations in mood. Setting up a system of regular visits and phone calls from doctors, social workers, family members, and friends is one option. It may be necessary to inform your boss or a colleague at work about your illness so they can catch early warning signs.

Educating yourself about some of the behavioral changes that occur when moods shift is a way to become more self-reliant. However, if you suspect a change in your mood, call someone. It can be difficult to pinpoint identifying factors, because many common emotions span several mood states, including euthymia (feeling good), depression, and hypomania. Signs of an incipient change may include the sudden appearance of irritability and anger or a disrupted night's sleep. Discussing how you feel and your recent activities with others may help you forestall the adverse effects of a full-blown mood swing. Do not make any changes in medication or therapy schedules yourself, even if you suspect it will help a mood swing.

Keep in mind that everyone's moods vary to some extent. It is a sustained change in mood over time—days and weeks, for example—that is critical to track.

How important is it for people with bipolar disorder to maintain a schedule of regular activity and wakefulness?

This is one of the most important factors for bipolar patients when trying to manage their illness. Life often seems disorganized and out of control for many bipolar patients. A firm, but not confining, daily structure allows them room to move within prescribed boundaries that help to ensure their safety and continued good health.

An ideal day would be as follows:

- getting up at the same time every morning (e.g., somewhere between 7:30 and 8:00 A.M.)
- dressing for work and having breakfast
- taking any medications that your doctor has prescribed for the morning
- going to work for a few hours
- taking a leisurely lunch hour, which may include a nap or meditation
- leaving work at nearly the same time each day
- having dinner with family or friends
- reading, taking a bath, or playing a game before bed
- taking any medications prescribed for the evening
- going to bed around the same time each night

Obviously, sticking to the same schedule every day is not always possible. Unexpected and unscheduled events arise, such as traffic jams and last-minute social plans. It is important not to be too rigid and to realize your limitations and not become overstimulated. For people with bipolar disorder, anxiety, stress, and alterations in sleep patterns are likely to induce mood swings. If you find it hard to maintain a schedule of regular activity, ask your doctor, parent, spouse, or a friend to help you modify your schedule to better fit your needs. Changing certain routines, even finding a new job, may make all the difference.

Should people with bipolar disorder limit the amount of stimulation and stress in their lives?

Definitely. For many people, a diagnosis of bipolar disorder means they have to reassess their career, school, and lifestyle choices. Edward, a fifty-three-year-old book editor who has lived with bipolar disorder for fifteen years, significantly reduced his workload. At one point, he was in charge of a very successful imprint at a large publishing house, but the pressure and stimulation were simply too intense. He lessened the stress in his life by cutting back to a three-day workweek and by working out of a quiet, suburban office near his home. He discovered that he often became more hypomanic after noisy, crowded office parties where he would sometimes have a number of drinks. He stopped going to the parties, thereby eliminating a stimulus that produced hypomanic symptoms.

Many bipolar patients react adversely to too much light, noise, and pressure. Establishing a low-pressure, nondistracting work environment and a peaceful home life are good ways to decrease the risk of both manic and depressive episodes. It is not easy reducing the stimulus level in a person's life, especially when the individual craves excitement and risk when hypomanic and manic. Anticipating what events and circumstances might provoke a manic or depressive episode is a fundamental coping task for doctors, patients, and their families.

How does an early diagnosis affect lifestyle choices?

If a person is diagnosed during his preteen, adolescent, or early-adulthood years, the diagnosis may influence choices about schooling and career. Anticipating, planning, and possibly lowering certain expectations this early in a person's life can seem limiting, but it may mean a markedly better prognosis. Conversely, many bipolar patients do reach their life goals and learn to cope with stress *without* having to lower their expectations.

For the newly diagnosed patient who has shown some behavioral problems in the past, choosing a low-stress school environment is almost always the right choice. Schools that do not impose strict time limits and have fewer academic pressures than more competitive ones tend to be optimal. Nevertheless, the school should still have an established structure for students that makes them feel secure and capable. Doctors and parents should take great care not to make the young person feel as though he will have to lead a compromised or stigmatized life. Generally this is not the case.

If someone is diagnosed with bipolar disorder at an early age, do they miss certain developmental landmarks?

Individuals who are diagnosed with bipolar disorder in their teen or early-adulthood years *may*, but certainly not always, be deprived of achieving certain developmental milestones at the usual time. These include separation from family and parents, sexual experimentation, development of intimate relationships, rejection, higher education, marriage, child bearing, child rearing, and career opportunities. For many people with bipolar disorder, these developments are delayed or impaired. Psychotherapy offers patients a setting to discuss missing certain milestones at developmentally appropriate ages. Recovering lost time is impossible, but patients can learn to experience transitions and new relationships at their own pace. Keep in mind that it is often these very developmental transitions that can induce episodes of both depression and mania.

Is career counseling recommended for people with bipolar disorder?

Sometimes it becomes necessary for bipolar patients to modify their career choices and lifestyles after they have been diagnosed. You may not experience immediate results, but it will probably make a big difference over time. Career counselors can recommend certain professional pathways that may help to alleviate pressure without greatly limiting a person's choices. Ironically, many people with bipolar disorder seek high-paced careers and crave stimulating lifestyles. They must learn to limit their expectations and nurture a work and home life that will be more conducive to stable moods.

Are there any ways I can learn to identify the early signs of hypomania?

It is not easy to catch oneself becoming hypomanic, because, as mentioned before, the symptoms feel good. However, there are some ways that you or another person can identify when you might be in the early stages of a mood swing.

Two techniques for identifying hypomanic symptoms are:

1. *The two-person rule:* The person agrees to discuss new ideas and plans with two trusted people. This allows for a period of taking stock and reflection.

2. *Activity scheduling:* The goal here is to regulate daily activities with the hope of keeping a person's mood stabilized. The fewer unknowns there are in the daily routine, the less chance there is for symptomatic behavior.

What are some ways I can potentially prevent a hypomanic or manic episode?

Preventing hypomanic and manic episodes is not always possible, but there are ways to calm yourself down if you feel as if your mood is changing. Some of these ways are:

• When you are in an overstimulating situation (e.g., a party, a rock concert, or a family argument), literally remove yourself. Leave the party, go outside for some air, or go to another room and close the door.

• Meditation is a useful technique for limiting external stimulation. It may not always be possible in the middle of the day to close out the rest of the world in order to meditate. Sitting in a bathroom stall or in a quiet office with the door closed may help to limit noise and intrusion.

• Asking family members and colleagues if they notice a change in your mood and behavior. For example:

Have you begun doing more work than usual? Are you staying up later? Are you suddenly more sociable than in the past?

• If you are exposed to an abundance of bright light, you may need to remove yourself. Discos, planetariums with light shows, fireworks displays, and rock concerts can all produce enough bright light to induce manic symptoms in bipolar patients. If possible, do not go alone to an event or performance where there will be bright lights.

Are there any substances I should avoid if I have bipolar disorder?

Throughout your treatment, you and your doctor will discuss what substances you should avoid. Generally, you should not ingest or inject anything that can potentially alter brain chemistry or interfere with other physiologic functions. There is also the danger of adverse interactions with the medications you are taking. Some well-known substances to avoid include:

1. Caffeine
2. Alcohol
3. Cocaine
4. Marijuana
5. Any mood-altering drugs, herbs, and hormones
6. Decongestants and combination allergy medications

How can my family help me cope with bipolar disorder?

First, you must be willing to include them in your treatment. This is not to say that your family has to know everything about what you discuss with your doctor and what goes on in your psychotherapy sessions. They should know enough about bipolar disorder in general and your specific needs to help when necessary. Psychoeducation is just as important for them as it is for you. At certain times, your doctor may recommend family therapy to help resolve issues that are holding you back or causing you undue stress. If you are planning any large-scale changes in your life, like switching jobs, getting married, or moving to another city, it is important for you to inform your family.

In addition to emotional support, parents, spouses, siblings, and grown children can:

- remind patients to take their medications
- make sure that they do not miss doctor and psychotherapy appointments
- help keep life chart information up-to-date and pertinent
- be alert to any alteration in mood or behavior
- minimize the stigma of having a mental illness by educating others
- help create realistic education, career, and lifestyle choices

Do not forget to remind your family that you do not blame them for your illness, as guilt can be one of many factors that inhibit productive familial relationships. It is important for families to view their relatives with bipolar disorder as productive individuals whom they do not need to fawn over. If families are too lenient, bipolar relatives can develop an inappropriate sense of entitlement and dependency. Limit-setting can be extremely comforting to those with bipolar disorder and tends to impart a sense of security in their often chaotic world. No family should assume that coping with bipolar disorder is easy or clearly defined. The therapeutic setting is probably the most productive milieu in which to develop coping and life-management skills for everyone.

What if my immediate family is unable or unwilling to help me?

We have stressed throughout the book that people with
bipolar disorder should not have to manage the illness
alone. Unfortunately, not everyone's immediate or even
extended family is willing or able to be involved. In
these cases, bipolar patients need the support of close
friends—a "surrogate" family, as it were. Friends can
be easier to relate to because they and the patient tend
not to engage in the same emotional conflicts as family
members. If the bipolar patient is unable to create a
network from friends, then self-help groups, local organizations, and national support groups are other excellent resources. Your doctor, a psychologist, or a clinical
social worker can help you find emotional care when
you feel lost and alone, as can self-help and support
groups.

What are some general coping strategies for depression?

There are many coping mechanisms for people who are
trying to alleviate their depressive symptoms. Taking
medication is the most obvious, of course, but there are
also several behavioral and environmental factors that
can make you feel better. Do not overwhelm yourself
with too many coping skills at once. Try to choose an
activity that is relaxing and self-fulfilling, and that gives
you a more positive outlook on the world. If you have
trouble finding any pleasure or relief from the following
suggestions, talk to your doctor about modifying your
medication or psychotherapy schedule. Your depression
may be moving from mild to moderate to more severe,
and you and your doctor may need to reassess your
current condition.

COPING STRATEGIES FOR DEPRESSION

• *Medication:* Always stick to your medication schedule, whether you are taking mood stabilizers, antidepressants, or both.

- *Psychotherapy:* Try not to miss scheduled therapy appointments. If you are unable to make your session because you are sick or away, notify your therapist as soon as possible to schedule a telephone session or a makeup appointment.

- *Self-help and support groups:* As mentioned several times throughout this book, discussing your feelings with like-minded and open-minded people in a neutral setting can be very uplifting and enlightening.

- *Regular sleep patterns:* Some mornings you may feel so depressed that getting out of bed seems impossible. It is very common for depressed people to feel their worst in the morning. If this is the case for you, let yourself feel anxious, nervous, down-in-the-dumps, and sad if necessary. Allow time for lying in bed and contemplating what the day may bring. List the activities that will give you pleasure over the course of your day, and you may well discover the energy you need to push back the covers and get going. If you find it difficult to fall asleep or have restless nights, your doctor may be able to prescribe a sedative that will not interfere with your other medications.

- *Avoid stressful situations:* Stressful situations, like family arguments or frequent moves, are likely to increase both manic and depressive symptoms in bipolar patients. If you find that your depressive symptoms increase when you are faced with anxiety-producing events, you should know that you are not alone. You need to anticipate and avoid people and places that may make you more depressed and anxious. Working in therapy to minimize your exposure to particular conflicts with your immediate family is a good way to begin changing the dynamics that create stressful interactions. If pressure at work is more of a problem, you need to discuss with your employer and colleagues about modifying your duties and responsibilities. Similarly, you may need to reassess both romantic relationships and friendships if they are a source of stress that aggravates your condition.

• *Try not to be alone:* When alone, some people dwell more on depressing thoughts and the negative aspects of their lives. If you live alone but crave companionship and conversation, participate in local evening activities. Most cities have organizations, like the YMCA or YWCA, that offer lectures, films, concerts, workshops, and classes for both members and nonmembers. Joining a health club or a local sports team is a good way to meet people, stop thinking about your problems, and get some exercise to boot. Universities and libraries also offer diverse and fulfilling evening and weekend programs that tend to attract thoughtful and sensitive participants.

• *Set realistic expectations for the day:* Do not overload your daily schedule with unrealistic goals. If you do not meet all of your goals, you are likely to start beating yourself up and feeling more depressed. At the beginning of the day, choose one or two projects that you would like to focus on and stick to them. If you do not complete a proposal at work, a paper at school, or all the housework, do not be too hard on yourself. There is always tomorrow.

• *Avoid movies, books, and plays with upsetting subjects:* Most people find certain subjects particularly upsetting to them. Watching an extremely violent film or reading a book about a devastating war can make you feel worse rather than better. Often the evening news broadcast or daily newspaper can be too much for a depressed person. Wait until you are less depressed, or avoid disturbing material altogether even if other people recommend it. Learn what you can tolerate and use your judgment.

• *Attend cultural events that make you happy:* Just as some subjects make you depressed, others tend to lift your spirits and give you hope. Art, music, dance, and literature can have the ability to take you out of yourself for a brief period and make you forget how "blue" you are feeling. They can also offer perspective for those times when life seems pointless and dreary.

- *Take time off during the day:* All people have times during the day when they have more energy and enthusiasm than others. When you are feeling low or stressed, stop what you are doing and take some time to relax and gather your thoughts. Try to schedule your day around your peaks and valleys, setting aside time to engage in pleasurable and fulfilling activities that boost your mood.

- *Do not put pressure on yourself to be friendly and outgoing:* Your friends and family will understand if you are more reticent than usual. Almost everyone can empathize with someone who is feeling sad and blue, even if they do not understand the extent of your depression. Do not feel obligated to explain yourself to others if they encourage you to just "snap out of it." You owe no one an explanation, but you may want a friend or relative to explain to others what you are going through.

- *Attend religious services:* Going to church or synagogue, praying, and feeling part of a community are often quite beneficial for many depressed people. Realizing that you are not alone in your search for meaning and need for human contact can be very comforting and life-affirming.

- *Volunteer at a soup kitchen or local hospital:* Helping the less fortunate can make depressed individuals feel fulfilled and hopeful. Most nonprofit organizations, religious institutions, libraries, and hospitals are more than willing to accept volunteers.

- *Stay away from alcohol and drugs not prescribed by your doctor:* Alcohol is a depressant and can adversely interfere with bipolar medications in a variety of ways. Common recreational drugs, like cocaine and marijuana, as well as prescription medications can also impinge on bipolar treatments. Alcohol and drugs certainly have the ability to make you more depressed and may even induce mania in certain patients. Frankly, it is best to avoid them altogether if you have bipolar disorder.

• *Avoid making major life decisions:* Mild, moderate, and severe depression colors your perspective on your life. Relationships and work may seem unfulfilling and meaningless, and you may think change will make you happier. You may decide you want a divorce or want to quit your job in the midst of a depressive episode. Before you make any decisions or take any action, talk to your doctor and your family. They can offer a point of view that is not affected by depression and help you to see the larger picture.

• *The Internet:* The Internet is a useful tool for finding others who are coping with bipolar depression. Search for a chat room that puts you in touch with others and helps you to further your education about the disorder.

• *Self-care and nutrition:* Do not neglect your physical health. Make sure to eat regularly scheduled nutritious meals, but indulge with a favorite snack from time to time. Share home-cooked meals with friends and family. Treat yourself to a day at a spa that includes massage, aromatherapy, and meditation. If you are concerned that some spa activities might affect your bipolar medication, such as a Jacuzzi, a sauna, or a steam room, ask your doctor what she recommends.

• *Laugh each day:* Laughing is great for lifting spirits. Add a little humor to your daily routine by renting a funny movie, reading the comics, or watching your favorite stand-up comedian.

• *Play with children and animals:* Both children and animals can be quite life-affirming. They share qualities of wonder and innocence that can inspire, reduce stress, and lift your mood. If you have the energy to play a simple game with a child or take a dog for a walk, you may find that you feel better afterward.

Can I have bipolar disorder and feel like a normal person?

There are times when none of us feel "normal." We all perceive the world in our own way and draw on our inner and outer resources to cope with life's ups and downs. People with bipolar disorder may experience the "highs" and "lows" more intensely than others, but in between they also have long periods of normal functioning. Medication, alternate therapies (e.g., ECT), and psychotherapeutic treatments for bipolar disorder are becoming more refined and sophisticated with each passing year. Additionally, the overall understanding of the illness has never been greater and continues to increase steadily with dissemination of information over the Internet and through books and articles. Holding on to hope and staying in control are two of the greatest challenges for those with bipolar disorder. Knowing that help is available from countless resources is the first step toward leading a healthy, productive, happy, and "normal" life.

Glossary

Acupuncture: an ancient form of Chinese medicine in which specific points on the body are stimulated by hair-thin needles to restore the normal flow of bio-energy, or "qi"

Anticonvulsants: medications used for seizure disorders and, more recently, bipolar disorder; medications include Depakote, Tegretol, Neurontin, and Lamictal

Antidepressants: drugs designed to alleviate depressive symptoms by altering certain chemicals in the brain and changing brain function

Antimanic Medication: drugs used to stabilize mood in manic patients; medications include lithium, Depakote, Tegretol, and others

Antipsychotic Medication: drugs designed to calm a psychotic patient; medications include Clozaril, Thorazine, and Haldol

Attention Deficit Hyperactivity Disorder (ADHD): a disorder commonly diagnosed in children, but also prevalent in adults, that is marked by an inability to concentrate and focus, and hyperactivity

Atypical Neuroleptics: medications that are part of a group of antipsychotic drugs known as neuroleptics; they include Clozaril, Zyprexa, and Risperdal

Benzodiazepines: antianxiety drugs; they include Klonopin and Ativan

Bilateral ECT: an electroconvulsive therapy technique that uses electrodes placed on both temples of the head

Bipolar Disorder: episodes of clinical depression (lasting at least two weeks) and periods of hypomania (lasting at least four days) or mania (lasting at least one week); also known as manic depression or manic-depressive illness

Bipolar I Disorder: a form of the disorder marked by significant periods of mania and various degrees of depression

Bipolar II Disorder: a form of the disorder marked by significant depressions and hypomania (milder form of mania)

Bipolar III Disorder: an unofficial diagnosis given to a patient who is generally depressed and becomes manic when taking antidepressant medication; a family history of depression is also present

Breakthrough Episode: when a patient develops symptoms of mania or depression even when on medication

Brief Psychotherapy: any psychotherapeutic modality that focuses on a specific goal and is concluded over several weeks to one year of therapy sessions

Calcium Channel Blockers: usually used for treating hypertension; affects the movement of calcium into cells of the heart and blood vessels; medications such as Nimotop and Calan may have antimanic properties

Circadian Rhythms: the "internal clock" that sets an individual's daily schedule; natural rhythm of sleep and wakefulness

"Clang" Association: clinical term used to describe a patient who rhymes words in a free-associative thought pattern

Classical Psychoanalysis: a form of psychotherapy developed by Sigmund Freud that focuses on a patient's childhood, personality development, and unconscious; patient usually has several sessions each week over a period of many years

Cognitive Distortions: inappropriately negative or "skewed" thoughts that may lead to a distorted sense of self, low self-esteem, and poor functioning

Cognitive-Behavioral Psychotherapy: a form of psychotherapy that helps patients identify negative thought patterns and change them into positive ones

Comorbid Disorder: where two or more diseases coexist at the same time

Complete Blood Count (CBC): a measurement of red and white blood cells; useful in detecting anemia, infections, allergies, and other disorders

Convulsion: repetitive overfiring of brain neurons, which leads to various forms of sensory and motor changes; also known as a seizure

Cross-Sectional Issues: relates to the immediate concerns of a depressive or manic episode

Cyclothymic Disorder: repeated episodes of mild depressions and mild manias

Delusion: extreme false belief

Denial: a person's unconscious inability to accept reality and cope with it

Depression: a mood disturbance marked by sadness, pessimism, hopelessness, and related feelings coupled with a lack of interest or loss of pleasure; subject of another book in this series: *If You Think You Have Depression*

Depression Scale: a psychological questionnaire designed to detect the presence or severity of depression (e.g., Beck Depression Inventory)

Depressive Episode: an episode that meets the criteria for a major depressive episode lasting at least two weeks; features include depressed mood, loss of interest in pleasurable activities, sleep disturbance, and loss of appetite

Dopamine: one of several brain chemicals, or neurotransmitters, believed to play a role in controlling mood

Dysthymia: a mild, chronic depression or despondency that lasts for at least two years in adults and one year in children and adolescents

Dysthymic Disorder: see *dysthymia*

Electroconvulsive Therapy (ECT): a treatment for severe depression and bipolar disorder that produces brief, generalized seizures by passing an electrical current through the brain

ECT Suite: room where a physician performs electroconvulsive therapy

Electrocardiogram (EKG): the tracing made by an electrocardiograph machine that monitors heart activity

Electroencephalogram: a machine that monitors brain-wave activity

Emil Kraepelin: German psychiatrist who established, among other things, criteria for manic-depressive illness that is still used today for diagnosing bipolar I disorder

Family Therapy: a type of psychotherapy that enables families to discuss issues, learn how family dynamics affect patients, and work together to treat patients more effectively

First Messenger System: a process whereby neurotransmitters hook up with receptors on the outside of brain cells

fMRI: a type of brain imaging that allows for observation and study of brain function in specific areas

Gaba-Aminobutryic Acid (GABA): a brain chemical known as the "quieting" neurotransmitter because of its calming effects

Genetic Counseling: a form of counseling for people with medical and psychological concerns and questions regarding reproduction and inheritance of diseases

Grief: a period of normal sadness and melancholia that generally occurs after the loss of a loved one or thing

Group Therapy: a therapeutic setting in which a small group of individuals exchange information and ideas relating to their condition with the aid of trained professionals, usually a psychiatrist, psychologist, and/or a clinical social worker

Growth Hormone: also known as somatotropin; this hormone is necessary for bone and cartilage growth

Hallucination: extreme false perception (e.g., hearing voices)

Heterocyclic Antidepressant: an antidepressant with a variable-ringed molecular structure (e.g., Asendin)

Hypericum Perforatum: see *St. John's wort*

Hypersomnia: oversleeping

hyperthyroidism: an overactive thyroid gland, often caused by an autoimmune disorder resulting in an overproduction of thyroid hormones; symptoms may mimic mania or depression

Hypnotherapy: a psychotherapeutic modality that places the patient in a state of relaxed wakefulness and heightened concentration

Hypomania: a mild form of mania characterized by elevated, elated, or irritable mood, optimism, decreased need for sleep, and abundance of energy

Hypomanic Episode: symptoms that meet the criteria for a hypomanic episode are similar to those for a manic episode; they are not severe enough to cause marked impairment in social and professional functioning; must last at least four days

Hypothyroidism: an underactive thyroid gland causing an underproduction of thyroid hormones; symptoms may mimic depression

Informed Consent: an agreement drawn up by a patient and doctor whereby the patient is explained the risks and benefits of a specific medical intervention

Insomnia: sleep difficulty

Interpersonal Psychotherapy: a form of psychotherapy that focuses on conflicts, distortions, and difficulties that people have in their relationships with others

Kindling: small electrophysiological impulses in the brain that create low-level disruptions which can lead to full-blown seizures

Life Charts: charts and graphs that patients use to track moods, activities, life events, and the course of their illness

Light Therapy: also known as phototherapy, exposure to bright light in order to relieve symptoms of seasonal affective disorder; may induce mania in some bipolar patients

Limbic System: sometimes called the emotional center of the brain or the emotional brain; handles emotional and social functioning such as family attachment and falling in love

Maintenance Medication: medication taken to prevent onset of possible future manic and depressive episodes; usually a mood stabilizer; can include antianxiety or antidepressant agents

Major Depressive Disorder: a depressed mood or loss of interest or pleasure plus other symptoms that last over a period of two or more consecutive weeks; other symptoms may include significant weight loss, sleep disturbance, concentration difficulties, fatigue, and low self-esteem

Mania: a mood disturbance marked by an abnormally elevated, expansive, or irritable mood, racing thoughts, pressured speech, sleep disturbance, grandiose feelings, distractibility, and poor judgment

Manic Depression or Manic-Depressive Illness: see *bipolar disorder*

Manic Episode: an episode that meets the criteria for mania over a period of at least one week; patient must exhibit at least four symptoms for mania

Meditation: a stress-reduction technique of quietly focusing on the breath, a word, or an action in order to bring the physical, mental, and emotional states into balance; participants are encouraged to "empty" their minds while meditating

Melatonin: a central nervous system hormone secreted by the pineal gland; used most commonly for jet lag; may have implications in the treatment of depression

Milieu Therapy: an ambient therapeutic environment that exists in a psychiatric hospital, outpatient unit, or clinic

Mixed Mood Episode: a diagnosis that is made when symptoms of depression and mania occur simultaneously almost every day for a period of time lasting at least one week

Monoamine Oxidase Inhibitors (MAOIs): a class of antidepressants that inhibit an enzyme that breaks down norepinephrine, thus making more of the neurotransmitter available in the brain

Mood Center: a collection of different neurons spread throughout the brain that control mood

Mood Disorder: a psychiatric diagnosis that includes depression, dysthymia, bipolar disorder, and mania

Mood Stabilizer: a drug that blocks both manic and depressive symptoms—for example, lithium, valproate (Depakote), or carbamazepine (Tegretol)

Neuron: brain cell

neurotransmitter: a chemical messenger that facilitates communication between brain cells

Norepinephrine: a brain chemical, or neurotransmitter, believed to play a role in controlling mood

Novel Antidepressants: see *heterocyclic antidepressants*

Observing Ego: the intellectual part of the psyche that can take a step back and look at life objectively even when emotions are in turmoil

Occupational Therapy: a form of therapy that enables patients to learn the everyday skills they need to take care of themselves out of a hospital or inpatient setting

Omega-3 Fatty Acids: a class of polyunsaturated lipids found in fish oil; may have potential as a mood stabilizer

Phototherapy: see *light therapy*

Placebo Effect: a positive or negative effect of a drug that stems from a person's expectations rather than the drug's active ingredient

Pluralistic Psychotherapy: a form of talking therapy that combines certain aspects of various psychotherapeutic techniques into one treatment

Postpartum "Blues": short period of tearfulness that occurs one to five days after delivery and usually resolves itself without treatment in a few days

Postpartum Depression: symptoms of major depression that begin within a year of giving birth and last at least two weeks

Premenstrual Dysphoric Disorder: a condition in which a remarkably depressed mood, marked anxiety, and decreased interest in activities regularly occur during the week leading up to menses and remitting within a few days after the onset of menstruation

Primary Insomnia: difficulty falling asleep

Psychiatrist: a medical doctor who specializes in the treatment of psychiatric illnesses and conditions; M.D. follows the name

Psychoeducation: a form of psychotherapy that teaches patients and their families about psychiatric illnesses and how to cope with them

Psychologist: a specialist in the use of psychotherapeutic techniques to treat mental disorders; Ph.D. or Psy.D. follows the name

Psychomotor Agitation: the visible speeding up of body movements and physical reactions; extreme nervousness

Psychomotor Retardation: the visible slowing down of body movements and physical reactions

Psychopharmacologist: a psychiatrist or other medical doctor who is an expert in medications used to treat psychiatric disorders

Psychosocial Therapy: a form of therapy that aims to teach patients the social skills they may lack to function normally in society

Psychosomatic Illness: any in a range of physical symptoms that can be attributed to a mental, rather than a physical, cause; also known as psychophysiological disorder

Psychotherapist: a trained professional who uses psychological methods to help people overcome or cope with mental illness; usually a psychiatrist, psychologist, or social worker; also known as "therapist"

Psychotherapy: a talking treatment for mental and emotional disorders using psychological methods

psychotic features: delusions, hallucinations, or other disruptions of perception that accompany manic or depressive symptoms

Psychotropic Drug: a medication that alters mood or otherwise affects the mind; mood stabilizers and antidepressants are psychotropic drugs

Rapid Cycling: four or more mood episodes (depressive, manic, or hypomanic), which may or may not alternate with each other, during a twelve-month period

Receptor: an area on the surface of a brain cell where chemical messengers (neurotransmitters) attach

Recreational Therapy: medically approved activities for inpatients; can include dramatics, sports, and visual arts

Refractory: when a medication stops working for a patient

Repetitive Transcranial Magnetic Stimulation (rTMS): an

experimental bipolar treatment in which a handheld coil generates a magnetic field that is passed through the head to create a small, localized electrical current in the brain

Seasonal Affective Disorder (SAD): a form of depression caused by changing light cues that occur in the late fall and winter; subject of another book in this series: *If You Think You Have Seasonal Affective Disorder*

Second Messenger System: an explosion of intercellular events that trigger DNA to make changes in brain cells to control mood

Secondary Insomnia: waking up repeatedly during the night

Seizure: see *convulsion*

Selective Serotonin Reuptake Inhibitors (SSRIs): a class of antidepressants that increase the availability of serotonin in the brain; they include Celexa, Luvox, Paxil, Prozac, and Zoloft

Serotonin: one of several brain chemicals, or neurotransmitters, believed to play a role in controlling mood

Shock Treatment: see *electroconvulsive therapy*

Specifier: a term used to fine-tune a broad diagnosis of bipolar disorder or other mood disorder—for example, "psychotic features," "melancholic features," or "postpartum onset"

St. John's Wort: a yellow, flowering plant that is being studied in the United States as a treatment for mild to moderate depression; effects on bipolar disorder unknown

Supportive Psychotherapy: a form of talking therapy that focuses on the here and now; the therapist provides a great deal of guidance, advice, and direction

Tertiary Insomnia: waking up earlier than usual in the morning

Tetracyclic Antidepressants: an antidepressant with a four-ringed molecular structure (e.g., Wellbutrin)

Therapeutic Alliance: the conscious, working relationship that develops between a psychotherapist, patient, and sometimes the patient's family in order to treat and cope with an illness

Therapist: see *psychotherapist*

Thought Disorder: a general term that applies to anyone having problems expressing, conceptualizing, continuing, or abstracting a coherent thought

Traditional Psychodynamic Psychotherapy: a psychoanalytic modality that looks at the unconscious, early-childhood-development, and personality patterns related to a current mental problem

Tricyclic Antidepressants (TCAs): an antidepressant with a three-ringed molecular structure (e.g., Tofranil)

Unilateral ECT: electroconvulsive therapy technique using an electrode on one temple of the head; may produce less memory loss than bilateral ECT, but also may be less effective

Visualization: a therapy technique that uses symbolic images to help patients understand and cope with a medical or psychological condition

Vocational Therapy: helps patients identify and develop professional and academic skills in preparation for returning to work or school

Appendix A:

Resources

SUPPORT GROUPS

Keep in mind that while support groups can be an integral part of a treatment plan and enhance the quality of a person's life, they are not a substitute for medication and psychotherapy. Do not take any medical advice from a nonprofessional without first consulting with your own doctor.

**National Depressive and Manic-Depressive
    Association**
730 North Franklin Street, Suite 501
Chicago, IL 60610
800–826–(DMDA) 3632 or 312–642–0049
Internet address: http://www.ndmda.org/

Founded 1986. Provides support and information for patients and families and public education on the biochemical nature of depressive illnesses. Annual conferences, chapter development guidelines, newsletter.

Depression and Related Disorders Association
Meyer 3–181, 550 bldg.
600 North Wolfe Street
Baltimore, Maryland
410–955–4647
Internet address: http://infonet.welch.jhu.edu/
    departments/drada/default/

Founded 1987. Provides educational materials to sufferers, their families, and the general public. Also gives out information regarding local and national support groups.

> **Madison Institute of Medicine (formerly the
>   Lithium Information Center)**
> 7617 Mineral Point Road
> Madison, WI 53717
> 608–827–2470
> (fax) 608–827–2479

Founded 1975. Has an extensive physicians' referral and support group list and information regarding specialist services for physicians, patients, and families. Will perform a search and provide articles for a nominal fee.

> **National Foundation for Depressive Illness**
> P.O. Box 2257
> New York, NY 10016
> 800–239–1295

An informal service that provides a recorded message of the clear warning signs of depression and bipolar disorder, and instructs how to get help and further information. For a bibliography and referral list of physicians and support groups in your area, send $5 and a self-addressed, stamped business-size envelope with 98 cents postage.

> **Mood Disorders Support Group, Inc.**
> P.O. Box 1747
> Madison Square Station
> New York, NY 10159
> 212–533–MDSG (6374)

Founded 1981. Provides support and education for people with bipolar disorder or depression and their families and friends. Guest lectures, newsletters, rap groups, assistance in starting groups.

Bipolar Network News
c/o Stanley Foundation
5430 Grosvenor Lane, Suite #200
Bethesda, MD 20814
800–518–7326

Offers a free subscription to Bipolar Network News [a joint project with the National Alliance for the Mentally Ill (NAMI) and National Institute of Mental Health (NIMH)]. Provides a physician referral service, outreach, information on clinical drug trials, early-intervention programs for children.

Depressed Anonymous
P.O. Box 17414
Louisville, KY 40217
502-459-6700

Founded 1985. Twelve-step program to help depressed persons believe and hope they can feel better. Newsletter, phone support, information, referrals, pen pals, workshops, conference, seminars. Information packet ($5), group starting manual ($10.95).

Association for the Advancement of Behavior
    Therapy
305 Seventh Avenue, 16th floor
New York, NY 10001
212–647–1890 or 800–685–AABT (2228)

Founded 1966. A membership organization for therapists, researchers, and academics. Excellent for anyone interested in the teaching and practice of cognitive-behavioral therapy (CBT). Publishes reference material for members; offers peer reviews, newsletter, annual conference. For the general public, provides a list of therapists who use CBT in any given state. For a nominal fee, will perform search. As of December 1, 1998, will have a Web-based reference directory for general public to search for participating doctors. Internet address: www.aabt.org./aabt

Depression After Delivery
P.O. Box 1282
Morrisville, PA 19067
800–944–4773 or 215–295–3994
Internet address: http://www.behavenet.com/dadinc

Founded 1985. Provides support and information for women who have suffered from postpartum depression. Telephone support in most states, newsletter, group development guidelines, pen pals, conferences.

National Organization for Seasonal Affective
    Disorder
(NOSAD)
P.O. Box 40190
Washington, DC 20016
(no phone)

Founded 1988. Provides information and education on the causes, natures, and treatment of seasonal affective disorder. Encourages development of services to patients and families, research into causes, and treatment. Newsletter.

SELECTED WEB SITES

http://www.psycom.net/depression.central.html
http://www.mentalhealth.com/p.20html
http://www.mentalhealth.com/dis/p20-md02.html
http://www.yahoo.com/Health/Mental_Health/
    Diseases_and_Conditions
http://www.sk.sympatico.ca/healthway/REV_HTML/
    R6724.html
http://www.mahidol.ac.th/mahidol/ra/rapc/
    mooddx.html

http://www.schizophrenia.com/ami/diagnosis/
   manicDep.html
http://www.frii.com/parrot/bip.html

PROFESSIONAL ORGANIZATIONS

American Psychiatric Association
1400 K Street, N.W.
Washington, DC 20005
phone: 202–682–6325
fax: 202–692–6255

American Psychological Association
750 First Street, N.E.
Washington, DC 20002–4242
202–336–5500

American Society of Clinical Psychopharmacology
P.O. 2257
New York, NY 10116
212–268–4260

OTHER INFORMATION SERVICES

National Institute of Mental Health
D/ART (Depression Awareness, Recognition, and
   Treatment) Program
Room 15-C-05
5600 Fishers Lane
Rockville, MD 20857
800–421–4211
Internet address: http://www.nimh.nih.gov/

National public and professional education program
sponsored by the National Institute of Mental Health.
D/ART's goal is to alleviate suffering for the one in ten
American adults with depressive illnesses and is based
on more than fifty years of medical and scientific re-

search on depression. (Discussed further in chapter 4 of
this book.)

National Alliance for the Mentally Ill
200 North Glede Road, Suite 1015
Arlington, VA 22203–3754

National Institute of Mental Health
Division of Communications
5600 Fishers Lane
Rockville, MD 20857
301–443–4536

National Mental Health Association
1021 Prince Street
Alexandria, VA 22314–2971
703–684–7722

Appendix B:

Further Reading

A Brilliant Madness: Living with Manic-Depressive Illness, by Patty Duke and Gloria Hochman (Bantam Books, 1992).

Manic-Depressive Illness, by Frederick K. Goodwin, M.D. and Kay Redfield Jamison, Ph.D. (Oxford University Press, 1990).

An Unquiet Mind: A Memoir of Moods and Madness, by Kay Redfield Jamison, Ph.D. (Vintage Books, 1996).

Touched with Fire: Manic-Depressive Illness and the Artistic Temperament, by Kay Redfield Jamison, Ph.D. (Free Press, 1993).

Bipolar Disorder: A Family-Focused Treatment Approach, by David J. Miklowitz and Michael J. Goldstein (The Guilford Press, 1997).

A Mood Apart: The Thinker's Guide to Emotion and Its Disorders, by Peter C. Whybrow, M.D. (HarperPerennial, 1997).

For a more general view regarding depression, please refer to the following books:

Prozac and the New Antidepressants, by William S. Appleton (Plume, 1997).

How to Heal Depression, by Harold H. Bloomfield, M.D. and Peter McWilliams (Prelude Press, 1994).

Feeling Good: The New Mood Therapy, by David Burns, M.D. (Signet, 1980).

The Depression Workbook, by Mary Ellen Copeland (New Harbinger Publications, 1992).

On the Edge of Darkness: Conversations about Con-

quering Depression, by Kathy Cronkite (Doubleday, 1994).

Understanding Depression, by Donald Klein, M.D. and Paul Wender, M.D.—founders of the National Association for Depressive Illness (Oxford, 1993).

From Sad to Glad, by Nathan S. Kline, M.D. (Ballantine Books, 1991).

Undercurrents, by Martha Manning (HarperSanFrancisco, 1994).

Depression: The Mood Disease, by Francis Mark Mondimore (Johns Hopkins University Press, 1993).

Overcoming Depression, by Demitri F. and Janice Papolos (HarperPerennial, 1992).

The Beast: A Reckoning with Depression, by Tracy Thompson (Putnam, 1995).

You Are Not Alone, by Julia Thorne with Larry Rothstein (HarperCollins, 1993).

Prozac Nation: Young and Depressed in America, by Elizabeth Wurtzel (Houghton Mifflin Company, 1994).

Index